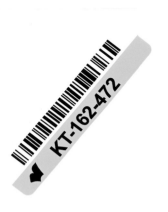
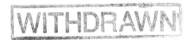
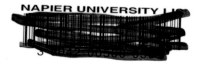

Springer Series on Geriatric Nursing

Mathy D. Mezey, RN, EdD, FAAN, Series Editor
New York University Division of Nursing

1992 Critial Care Nursing of the Elderly
   Terry T. Fulmer, RN, PhD, FAAN, and Mary K. Walker, PhD, RN, FAAN

1993 Health Assessment of the Older Individual, Second Edition
   Mathy Doval Mezey, RN, EdD, FAAN, Shirlee Ann Stokes, RN, EdD, FAAN, and Louise Hartnett Rauckhorst, RNC, ANP, EdD

1994 Nurse–Physician Collaboration: Care of Adults and the Elderly
   Eugenia L. Siegler, MD, and Fay W. Whitney, PhD, RN, FAAN

1995 Strengthening Geriatric Nursing Education
   Terry T. Fulmer, RN, PhD, FAAN, and Marianne Matzo, PhD(c), RN, Cs

Terry T. Fulmer, RN, PhD, FAAN is Professor of Nursing, New York University, and Director, Columbia University-New York Geriatric Education Center. She has held faculty appointments at the Columbia University School of Nursing, the Boston College School of Nursing, the Harvard Division on Aging, and the Yale School of Nursing. She is a gerontological nurse specialist with special expertise in elder abuse and acute care of the elderly. She lives in Rye, New York with her husband and 3 children.

Marianne Matzo, PhD(c), RN, CS, is Associate Professor of Nursing at New Hampshire Technical College at Manchester and a Doctoral Candidate at the University of Massachusetts/Boston Gerontology Institute. She is the former Gerontology Project Director at Saint Anselm College and has published extensively in the area of gerontological nursing education. Her research focuses on the areas of suicide among older adults and issues of productive aging.

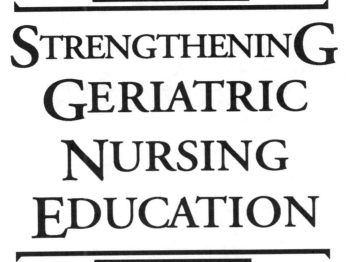

STRENGTHENING GERIATRIC NURSING EDUCATION

Terry T. Fulmer, RN, PhD, FAAN

Marianne Matzo, RN, PhD (cand.)

Editors

Springer Publishing Company

Copyright © 1995 by Springer Publishing Company, Inc.

Springer Publishing Company, Inc.
536 Broadway
New York, NY 10012-3955

Cover design by Tom Yabut
Production Editor: Pamela Ritzer

95 96 97 98 99 / 5 4 3 2 1

Library of Congress Cataloging-in-Publication Data

Strengthening geriatric nursing education / Terry T. Fulmer, Marianne
    Matzo, editors.
        p.   cm. — (Springer series on geriatric nursing)
    Includes bibliographical references and index.
    ISBN 0-8261-8940-7
    1. Geriatric nursing—Study and teaching.   I. Fulmer, Terry T.
II. Matzo, Marianne.   III. Series.
    [DNLM: 1. Geriatric Nursing—education.   2. Education, Nursing,
Graduate.   3. Education, Nursing, Continuing.   WY 18.5 S915 1995]
RC954.S78   1995
610.73'65'0711—dc20
DNLM/DLC
for Library of Congress   95-2116
                                                                    CIP

Printed in the United States of America

This book is dedicated to my husband, Keith, and our children, Nina, Holly, and Sam—who consistently support my efforts and keep me laughing. Special thanks to my mentor, Mathy Mezey, who always has time for everything.

Terry T. Fulmer

To my husband Roland for all of his love and support.
To my mentor, Dr. Lillian R. Goodman, for the insight and wisdom she has freely shared over the years.

Marianne Matzo

Contents

Contributors   ix

Foreword by Mark H. Beers, M.D.   xi

Preface by Terry T. Fulmer   xiii

Acknowledgment   xv

Part I   An Overview of Geriatric Nursing Education

1   Why Good Ideas Have Not Gone Far Enough:
    The State of Geriatric Nursing Education   3
    Mathy Mezey

2   Barriers in Nursing Education   21
    Marianne Matzo

3   Incorporating Geriatrics into the Licensure and
    Accreditation Process   29
    Terry T. Fulmer and Mary Tellis Nyack

4   Expanding Clinical Experiences   37
    May L. Wykle and Carol M. Musil

5   Student Resistance: Overcoming Ageism   49
    Carla Mariano

6   Integrated versus Course-Specific Programs   63
    Susan E. Sherman and Mary Burke

7 Lessons from Successful Curriculum Models   67
         Susan E. Sherman

Part II   Approaches to Specific Content Areas

8 Physiological Changes in Aging   77
         Mary Burke and Susan E. Sherman

9 Psychiatric Mental Health Content for
         Gerontological Nursing Education   85
         Carol M. Musil and May L. Wykle

10 Elimination and Skin Problems   99
         Marie O'Toole

11 Drugs and Their Side Effects   115
         Barbara K. Haight and Karen Cassidy King

12 Cancer and Pain Management for Elders:
         Recommendations for Nursing Curriculum   129
         Suzanne K. Goetschius

13 HIV and Older Adults   141
         Suzanne K. Goetschius

14 Teaching about Bioethics and the Elderly   153
         Mathy Mezey

15 On Vital Aging   161
         Betty Friedan

Appendix   169

Index   177

CONTRIBUTORS

Mary Burke, DNSc, RN, CANP
Assistant Professor
Georgetown University
School of Nursing
Washington, DC 20007

Betty Friedan
author of *The Fountain of Age*
c/o Simon and Schuster
New York, NY 10020

Suzanne K. Goetschius, MS, RNCS, GNP
Assistant Professor
Department of Technical Nursing
University of Vermont
Burlington, VT 05405

Barbara K. Haight, PhD, RN
Professor
Medical University of South Carolina
College of Nursing
Charleston, NC 29425

Karen Cassidy King, RN, MSN, ARNP
Assistant Professor
School of Nursing
University of Louisville
Louisville, KY 40292

Carla Mariano, RN, EdD
Associate Professor and Director
Advanced Education in Nursing Science
Master's Degree Programs
New York University Division of Nursing
New York, NY 10012

Mathy Mezey, RN, EdD, FAAN
Independence Foundation
Professor of Nursing Education
New York University Division of Nursing
New York, NY 10012

Carol M. Musil, PhD, RN
Assistant Professor of Nursing
Case Western Reserve University
Frances Payne Bolton School of Nursing
Cleveland, Oh 44106

Marie O'Toole RN, EdD
Assistant Professor
Teachers College
Columbia University
New York, NY 10027

Susan E. Sherman, MA, RN
Professor and Head
Department of Nursing
Community College of Philadelphia
Philadelphia, PA 19130

Mary Tellis-Nayak
Director, Long Term Care
Joint Commission
Oakbrook Terrace, IL 60181

May L. Wykle, PhD, RN, FAAN
Florence Cellar Chair, Professor of
   Gerontological Nursing
Associate Dean
Case Western Reserve University
Frances Payne Bolton School of
   Nursing
Cleveland, OH 44106

FOREWORD

The Merck Company Foundation is proud to have sponsored, in collaboration with the Columbia University School of Nursing, a conference to bring together leaders in nursing education to discuss gerontological education for nurses. That conference proved to be exciting and productive. It is now our hope that many more educators will participate in those discussions through this publication and that they will further the task of assuring that every nurse receives the education necessary to provide the best care to older persons.

Merck believes that better education in geriatrics and gerontology for all health professionals is critical to improve care of the elderly. Additionally, our "Partners for Healthy Aging" program provides comprehensive support for geriatrics both within Merck and to the greater health care community. We applaud the work done by those involved in producing this book and enthusiastically encourage those who read it to actively support the cause of gerontologic and geriatric education.

MARK H. BEERS, M.D.
Associate Editor of the Merck Manuals
Senior Director of Geriatrics
West Point, PA 19486

PREFACE

We are certainly indebted to the Merck Company Foundation for bringing together gerontological nursing educators from across the country to project the educational goals which will to take us into the next Century. Much progress has been made since the early 1960s when gerontological nursing was first thought of as a "subspecialty." Today, we can be proud of our gerontological nursing certification programs through the American Nurses Association, our basic Masters and Doctoral programs in gerontological nursing, and the continued progress in the realm of gerontological nursing research, which will ultimately produce our cutting-edge curricula.

In compiling this text, it is our sincere hope that it will outline some of the challenges we have yet to face. Without such self-examination, we have little hope of meeting the needs of the growing numbers of elderly in this country. It is our sincere hope that this text will be useful to educators across all levels of nursing programs who strive to create a curriculum that can ultimately improve care to older Americans.

Terry T. Fulmer

ACKNOWLEDGMENT

This book is derived from the conference, "Caring for Older Americans: The Critical Role of Nursing Education" sponsored by Columbia University School of Nursing Education Development Center, Inc., with the support of the Merck Company Foundation.

Part I

An Overview of Geriatric Nursing Education

Chapter 1

WHY GOOD IDEAS HAVE NOT GONE FAR ENOUGH: THE STATE OF GERIATRIC NURSING EDUCATION

Mathy Mezey

E vidence from practice in hospitals and long-term care facilities supports the conclusion that care delivered to elderly patients is far from ideal. In hospitals, elderly patients continue to be at risk for iatrogenic complications, use of physical restraints, and undiagnosed and untreated delirium. Recent studies call into question the quality and safety of shortened hospital lengths of stay. In nursing homes we still fail to individualize care, and concerns as to quality of care continue to surface in the lay and professional literature.

The extent to which failure in the education of nurses contributes to poor clinical outcomes for elderly patients is unknown. Attendees at the conference "Caring for Older Americans: The Central Role of Nursing Education" agreed that geriatric content should be a mandatory component of every nursing curriculum and that every nursing program should have at least one tenure-track faculty member certified in gerontological nursing.

Portions of this chapter are from "Contemporary geriatric nursing," by T. Fulmer and M. Mezey in W. R. Hazzard and E. L. Bierman, et al. (Eds.), *Principles of geriatric medicine and gerontology, 3e,* © 1994 McGraw-Hill, Inc. Reprinted with permission.

Unfortunately, we do not know whether nursing programs currently meet this standard. In fact, we know very little about the geriatric content in nursing programs. Faculty attending the conference said they need information about curriculum, faculty preparation, and students in geriatrics in order to plan curricula in geriatric nursing. This chapter summarizes what is and is not known about geriatrics in academic nursing programs, and speculates on why geriatric nursing has failed to gain a substantial toehold in nursing programs.

GERIATRICS IN NURSING EDUCATION: WHAT IS AND IS NOT KNOWN

It would be reasonable to assume that the increased number of elderly, the changing face of American health care, and substantial shifts in health policy and funding have substantially changed geriatric nursing education since 1975, yet we lack empirical knowledge as to what these changes might be.

Geriatrics in Programs Preparing Nurses for Beginning Clinical Practice

Associate degree, diploma, and baccalaureate programs provide nurses with basic preparation to function as generalists in ambulatory settings, home care, hospitals, and nursing homes. Irrespective of preparation, all new nurses sit for the same licensure examination to become RNs. Hospital-based diploma programs vary from two to three years in length, while associate-degree programs require two years of study in junior colleges or four-year universities. Baccalaureate programs, which in 1992 graduated over 50 percent of all new nurses, require four years of study in a college or university.[1]

The patterns of geriatric nursing education and the preparation, focus, and work of geriatric nurses are shown in Tables 1.1 and 1.2. Traditionally, basic nursing programs have included very little geriatric nursing content. Some have clinical rotations in nursing homes where students learn basic nursing skills: bathing, feeding, position-

TABLE 1.1 Preparation, Focus, and Work of Gerontological Nurses

License	Length of Preparation	Focus of Preparation	Primary Work Setting	Primary and Secondary Roles
Licensed practical nurse	12 months	Technical basic skills	Nursing home, MD's office, hospital	Technical (basic task nursing) work under supervision of RN
Registered nurse (ADN)	2 years	Entry level for basic technical nursing care	Hospital, nursing home, MD's office, home care	Direct patient care
Diploma	3 years	Entry level for basic care, technical and professional	Hospital, nursing home, MD's office, home care	Direct patient care
Baccalaureate (BSN, BS)	4 years	Entry level for professional nursing	Hospital, public health, home care, private practice	Direct patient care, supervisory position
Generic Master's (MSN)	2–3 years			
Nursing doctorate (ND)	3 years			
Master's (MS, MA, MN, MSN)	1–2 years	Advanced practice clinical specialist, nurse practitioner	Hospital, private practice, education, community-based agency	Expert clinical practice Specialty practice
Doctorate (PhD, DNSc)	3–7 years	Research, teaching, add to body of knowledge	School of nursing, federal/state agency	Teaching, research, policy, administration, clinical practice (independent or joint)

Source: Johnson, M. A., & Connelly, J. R.: Nursing and Gerontology: Status Report. Washington, DC, Association for Gerontology in Higher Education Advisory Committee on Nursing and Gerontology, 1990. Reproduced by permission.

TABLE 1.2 Patterns of Gerontological Nursing Education

	Undergraduate	Master's	Doctorate
Degree	ADN, diploma, BS, BA, BSN, generic master's, ND	MS, MN, MSN, MA	PhD, DNSc
Level	Entry level	Postbaccalaureate Clinical specialization	Post-master's
Focus	Generalist, beginning practitioner, "safe" practitioner	Functional role and leadership	Research, add to body of nursing knowledge or specialization
Method of entry	Licensure as RN	Graduation and/or advanced licensure certification (optional)	Graduation
Scope	Plan health care with elderly, use strengths of person, maximize capabilities, manage care	In-depth theory of aging Dynamics of aging Independent or collaborative practice Not setting-specific May be in two specialty areas: e.g., gerontology and administration	Public policy issues, clinical and theoretical research, independent or collaborative practice
Role	Registered nurse	GNP (clinician), GCNS, teacher administrator	Researcher, nurse executive, educator, practitioner
Course work	Medical–surgical, pediatrics, obstetrics, community mental health	Cognate, core (all master's), clinical-specific, functional role	Cognate, core, original scholarship

Source: Johnson, M. A., & Connelly, J. R.: *Nursing and Gerontology: Status Report.* Washington, DC, Association for Gerontology in Higher Education Advisory Committee on Nursing and Gerontology, 1990. Reproduced by permission.

ing patients. In hospital rotations, students primarily care for elderly patients. Unfortunately, because most faculty lack preparation in geriatric nursing, they focus on patients' general nursing and medical conditions rather than aspects of care—function and cognition, for example—that are the hallmark of geriatric practice.

More recently, however, several initiatives have supported the expansion of geriatric content in nursing programs. The W. K. Kellogg Foundation funded a national initiative, the Community College-Nursing Home Partnership, to prepare nursing students in associate-degree programs to work in nursing homes.[2] The six schools that participated in this project developed curriculum models that have been widely disseminated, and published competencies in geriatric nursing for students in associate, bachelors, and master's programs.

The impetus to increase geriatric content in baccalaureate programs has come from several sources. The Association for Gerontology in Higher Education has published recommendations related to outcomes and objectives for basic and advanced preparation in geriatric nursing and strategies for increasing geriatric content in nursing education.[3] The Teaching Nursing-Home Program, a national initiative funded by the Robert Wood Johnson Foundation, encouraged 11 baccalaureate schools of nursing to increase geriatric content in their curricula and to create clinical teaching sites for students in 12 affiliated nursing homes.[4,5] The project results indicate that, under favorable circumstances, students can have positive learning experiences in nursing homes. Over the course of the project, approximately 600 undergraduate students and over 300 graduate students had clinical rotations in the nursing homes. Undergraduate geriatric nursing for-credit course increased from 3 to 12; graduate courses doubled.[6]

The changing pool of applicants has also had a favorable effect on incorporation of geriatric content within schools of nursing. Increasingly, new applicants to nursing programs hold a second, and, at times, a third nonnursing degree.[7,8] The average age of students enrolled in baccalaureate programs in 1990 was 29 years.[7] Many baccalaureate programs encourage these mature students, and registered-nurse students, to accelerate their study toward a master's degree in nursing (BSN/MSN combined programs or generic masters' programs) or toward a nursing doctorate (ND), modeled after the JD and MD degrees. These students, many of whom have cared for elderly relatives, are sophisticated as to the changing demographics, enthusiastic about didactim (classroom) geriatric content, and often seek out clinical experiences with elderly patients.

Initiatives to improve the geriatric preparation of the generalist nurse have been further supported by the American Nurses Association (ANA) national certification process.[9] The ANA offers three levels of certification in gerontological nursing: gerontological nurse; geriatric nurse practitioner; and gerontological clinical nurse specialist. Certification as a gerontological nurse is open to all RNs, irrespective of academic preparation. Some schools of nursing encourage interested undergraduate students to prepare for this certification upon graduation. Nursing homes and hospitals wishing to upgrade nurses' geriatric skills offer courses that urge nurses to become certified as gerontological nurses.

While the aforementioned activities are encouraging, anecdotal evidence suggests that geriatric nursing continues to lag behind other areas of interest in generic nursing programs. We know of only a few baccalaureate programs that offer a required course in geriatric nursing. Even within the Teaching Nursing-Home Program, only 3 of the 11 participating schools had a required undergraduate geriatric nursing course.[6] When geriatric content is integrated into traditional medical and surgical nursing courses, which is most often the case, the quality of the content is very dependent on the preparation of the faculty teaching the course. Preparation of geriatric nursing faculty continues to be of grave concern. In one study where close to 60 percent of students' clinical experience involved patients 65 and over, less than 25 percent of faculty reported any preparation in care of the elderly.[10]

Geriatrics in Programs Preparing Nurses for Advanced Clinical Practice

Professional nurses wishing to specialize for advanced clinical practice complete a master's program that involves one to two years of full-time study. There are currently over 72,000 nurses with advanced clinical preparation. By the year 2000, the total supply is expected to reach 87,500, twice the 1988 supply.[11] Yet, this number will fall far short of the estimated need for 259,000 nurses with advanced clinical skills.[11,12]

University master's programs produce two streams of graduates prepared to assume advanced clinical positions: nurse practitioners and clinical specialists. Geriatric nurse practitioners (GNPs), geriatric clinical specialists (GNCs), and gero-psychiatric clinicians complete a formal educational program in care of the elderly and are certified for expanded practice by the American Nurses Association and/or state boards of nursing.[13]

The curriculum for most programs preparing nurses for advanced practice in geriatrics is based on the profession's Standards and Scope of Gerontological Nursing Practice,[14] the Standards of Practice for the Primary Health-Care Nurse Practitioner,[15] and the Clinical Specialist.[16] All programs teach physical, functional, and psychosocial assessment, physiology and pathophysiology, pharmacology, and recognition and management of physical and behavioral conditions associated with aging. Geriatric nurse practitioner and geriatric fellowship programs have been shown to teach similar content related to geriatric assessment.[17] While GNP programs are directed by nurse faculty, geriatricians, geriatric social workers, and other professionals participate in the presentation of content and supervision of students in clinical agencies.

In addition to didactic content, all programs require clinical rotations. Clinical practicums vary as to number of required hours; anecdotal data suggest that most programs require between 12 and 16 hours of practice per week.

In 1987, 37 academic programs prepared GNPs, 27 awarding advanced degrees and 10 providing continuing education certificates.[18] Both graduate and certificate programs average one year in length, and include both course work and clinical preceptorships.

In the 17 GNP programs currently funded by the Division of Nursing,[19] the average age of students is 31.5 years; 75 percent of students have four or more years of professional nursing experience prior to admission. After graduation, approximately 40 percent are employed either by nursing homes or by physicians with practices in nursing homes. Thirty five percent work in facilities in the inner city, and 20 percent in rural areas.

Preparation of GNPs and evaluation of their performance has received extensive support from the federal government and private foundations.[20,21] Since 1980, Congress has appropriated $1.3 million for the education of GNPs; the Veterans Administration has provided scholarships for candidates since 1982. Beginning in 1976, with funding from the Kellogg Foundation, the Mountain States Health Corporation educated, placed, and evaluated the effectiveness of 172 GNPs in over 200 nursing homes in 18 Western states.[22,23,24]

Less information is available about the preparation and number of geriatric clinical nurse specialists (GNCs) and gero-psychiatric clinical nurse specialists. The Division of Nursing currently funds 40 GNC programs.[18] Many GNCs, however, have prepared in adult clinical specialist programs that have electives or clinical options for gerontological specialization. There are currently three programs specifically preparing gero-psychiatric clinical specialists, but other programs preparing psychiatric nurse specialists also offer courses in gero-psychiatric nursing.[18] Three hundred nurses report a specialization in gero-psychiatric nursing.

The ANA offers national certification as either a GNP or GNC.[9] There is no certification examination for gero-psychiatric clinical nurse specialists.[9] Many states require certification by the ANA for recognition for advanced practice, including reimbursement. As of 1990, approximately 1200 GNPs were certified by the ANA. The total number of practicing GNPs, however, exceeds those with certification by the ANA, since some have prepared as adult and family nurse practitioners and others practice in states that use criteria other than that of the ANA to establish practice eligibility. The ANA certification for geriatric clinical nurse specialist was offered for the first time in 1991.[9]

Recognition of Advanced Practice Role

The federal government has extended third-party reimbursement for nurses with advanced preparation practicing in rural health settings (The Rural Health Act), and for dependents of military personnel through Civilian Health & Medical Program of Uniformed Services (CHAMPUS). As of 1992, Medicare, which had previously reim-

bursed for services provided by nurse midwives and nurse anesthe-
tists, extended reimbursement to GNPs and GNCs for services currently reimbursed to physicians for care of nursing-home residents.
Gero-psychiatric nurse specialists are not eligible for Medicare reimbursement. Designation of which nurses are eligible for such reimbursement is determined by each state through its nurse practice act.

All states have mechanisms for authorizing advanced nursing
practice, either through specific regulations by state boards of nursing (34 states), regulation by both boards of nursing and medicine
(eight states), or a broad nurse practice act permitting considerable
scope of practice (eight states).[25,26] Legislative authority to prescribe
has been granted to nurse practitioners in forty-eight states.[25,26]

Academic institutions are currently reassessing their preparation
of nurses for advanced practice. Nurse practitioners have traditionally been prepared to provide a broad range of direct services to
patients and families,[15,20,27,28,29] while clinical specialists are prepared
to provide primarily consultation and education about discrete clinical problems (i.e., renal disease, cancer, ostomy care) to patients,
families, and staff in hospitals.[16,30,31] Despite these distinctions, recent objective comparisons suggest striking similarities and very few
areas of difference in both the preparation and function of nurse
practitioners and clinical specialists, especially those in geriatric
practice. With the exception of pharmacology, GNP preparation
closely resembles that of GNCs.[32] Geriatric nurse practitioners and
GNCs often function interchangeably in hospitals, long-term care
facilities, and home care.[11] Newly passed legislation recognizes both
GNPs and GNCs as eligible for reimbursement under Medicare and
Medicaid.[25] In 1991, the ANA Councils of Clinical Nurse Specialists
and Primary Health Care Nurse Practitioners became one Council
of Advanced Nursing Practice. Thus, in the foreseeable future, GNP
and GNC preparation will in all likelihood merge into one program.

Gaps in Our Knowledge about Geriatric Content in Nursing Programs

While the preceeding section highlights what is known about geriatrics in nursing programs, there are, unfortunately, enormous gaps

in the existing knowledge base. Sorely needed is a national survey of the undergraduate and graduate curriculum, faculty, and graduates. Such a survey would provide specific knowledge as to 1) the current curriculum in geriatric nursing (course offerings, texts, hours of didactic and clinical content, types of clinical experiences, instruments, etc.); 2) the current preparation of faculty in geriatric nursing (education; research; publications; clinical practice; professional organization membership and activities, etc.); and 3) the graduates of master's programs in geriatric nursing (satisfaction with program, demographic information, type of practice before and after program completion).

SPECULATION AS TO WHY GERIATRICS HAS GAINED ONLY A PARTIAL TOEHOLD IN NURSING PROGRAMS

Despite the lack of a complete data base, there is substantial anecdotal evidence that geriatric nursing has, at best, achieved only a precarious toehold in academic nursing. Unfortunately, geriatrics does not appear to be integrated into the nursing curricula to the same degree as, for example, pediatrics or obstetrics.

While the absence of a sound data base makes speculation risky, we can identify six reasons for the failure of geriatrics to achieve full stature in academic nursing.

Failure to Clearly Articulate a Model for Practice with the Elderly That Would Guide Curriculum Development

Two competing models currently influence curriculum development:

1. Geriatric nursing as a primary-care specialty: In this model, geriatric nursing, like pediatrics, is a primary-care specialty in which nurses prepared at the advanced practice level (and geriatrician) develop practices in which they care for large numbers of elderly patients.

2. Geriatric nursing as a specialty, similar to neurological nursing or enterostomal therapists, etc.: In this model, geriatric nursing

is a referral specialty practice within medical surgical nursing. Most nurses would be expected to care for older people and thus would need basic knowledge in geriatrics. Only patients with diagnostic and treatment dilemmas are referred to geriatric nurse specialists (and geriatricians).

Failure to resolve these competing perspectives has tended to cloud curriculum development and has negative implications for the future integration of geriatrics in nursing education.

If geriatrics is a primary-care specialty, then there is not a great need to emphasize geriatrics in basic nursing programs (associate and baccalaureate). But if we were to adhere to this model, there would be a need to markedly expand advance practice preparation in geriatric nursing. This would suggest a separate course in geriatrics (similar to pediatrics and OB) at the associate and baccalaureate level taught by faculty prepared in geriatric nursing. We might allow undergraduate students wishing to work in geriatrics to take additional electives in geriatrics in their senior year. To meet primary-care demands, however, the most important educational implication would be to expand advanced practice programs (geriatric nurse practitioner programs) in geriatrics.

If, on the other hand, geriatrics is a typical referral specialty, then we need to assure that every student prepared in basic programs in nursing has minimal knowledge of care of the elderly and knows under what conditions to refer older patients to a nurse or physician "specialist." Such a model requires integration of a defined amount of geriatric content into every BSN and AD program. It would require only moderate expansion of GNP programs to meet specialty rather than primary-care needs, since such graduates would not be expected to deliver primary care.

Failure of Nursing Curricula to Reflect the Heterogeneity of the Elderly Population Seeking Care

Existing curricula have failed to reflect that the elderly comprise an extremely diverse group of people ranging in age from 65 to 95, a third of the lifespan.

In considering how best to integrate geriatrics, nursing faculty continue to engage in spurious discussions, for example, as to whether the focus of the curriculum should be on the well elderly (emphasizing prevention, etc.) versus the very frail elderly; whether beginning undergraduate students should have experiences in nursing homes, and whether caring for elderly patients in hospitals requires special knowledge. Nurse faculty also continue to be unclear about the degree to which older people need "protection," that is, whether they are a special population that need protection in terms of physical restraints and protection related to participation in research.[13]

Acknowledgment of the heterogeneity of the elderly population would have a marked impact on spreading geriatric content throughout the curriculum. For example, if there were agreement that health promotion of the elderly (promotion of sense of well being, immunizations, promotion of physical fitness, etc.) is required for all nursing students, then it could be integrated into a variety of courses regardless of setting.

Failure of the Curriculum to Address Intergenerational Issues in Care of the Elderly

Two examples serve to illustrate the failure of nursing programs to grasp the curricular opportunities related to intergenerational issues in geriatrics. In a recent discussion on curriculum content in community nursing and home care, nursing faculty failed to appreciate that the negative ramification of caring for elderly relatives or other family members needs to be included in course content in adult health and maternal–child health. Similarly, in a curriculum discussion related to a school-of-nursing-sponsored school-based clinic, faculty failed to appreciate that close to 60% of children in inner cities where this clinic is located are being raised by grandparents, many of whom are the *sole* guardians of these children.[33]

Full acknowledgment of the intergenerational issues related to care of the elderly would have important implications for infusing additional content related to the elderly in courses such as maternal–child and community-health nursing.

Unwillingness to Come to Grips with the Care of the Very Old and Frail Elderly

Nursing curricula continue to be driven by the paradigm of nursing homes as suspect and home care as always better than long-term institutional care. Despite the fact that 25% of people 45 and over will spend some time in a nursing home prior to death, nursing homes continue to be viewed as marginal institutions that offer, at best, limited educational opportunities. Moreover, leaders in geriatrics disagree conceptually as to whether nursing homes are primarily homes, hospitals, old-age centers, or something else.

Lack of conceptual clarity as to their purpose has impeded faculty from fully exploiting the training potential of nursing homes. It would behoove faculty to acknowledge the limitations of home care and reconceptualize nursing homes as integral components of the health-care continuum.

Failure to Create Models for Interdisciplinary Education

The literature is replete with examples of improvements in quality of care that can be achieved by geriatric teams.[34] Moreover, there is limited evidence that programs in geriatric nursing and medicine teach similar content related to assessment of elderly patients.[32]

Yet, within nursing education, examples of development of model, interdisciplinary training sites and courses are rare.[35] With a few notable exceptions, specifically within the Veterans Administration and in some geriatric education centers,[35] geriatric courses in nursing programs fail to adequately present didactic content in team development and lack clinical experiences in sites where practitioners practice as a team.

If nurses are to be prepared to practice alongside other professionals in caring for the elderly, they need to be exposed to interdisciplinary practice during their basic and advanced education. Such exposure should include both observation of how experienced professionals negotiate roles and also opportunities for direct involvement in interdisciplinary practice.

Failure to Prepare Adequate Numbers of Faculty in Geriatric Nursing

Faculty attending the conference from which this book is derived agreed that the days of "self-taught" gerontological nursing faculty are over. Nursing programs need faculty who have completed a formal program in geriatric nursing at the graduate level.

Although definitive numbers are not available, small studies show that most faculty currently teaching in nursing programs have very little or no preparation in care of the elderly. A recent survey in one academic nursing program found that while 70 percent of the patients taken care of by students were 65 and over, nursing faculty teaching adult health and illness had almost no preparation, either in for-credit or continuing-education courses, in geriatrics.[10]

Nursing curricula will continue to be deficient in geriatric content if faculty lack the knowledge, experience, and conviction that comes from specialized geriatric preparation. There is a critical need for both new and mid-career training of nurse educators.

CONCLUSION

While much is known, the most pressing need in geriatric nursing is for better data regarding how well nursing programs are doing in caring for older Americans. A second need is for a clearer and more accurate vision of who the elderly are, what are their needs, and how caring for older Americans impacts on the lives of all other Americans. A third critical need is for nursing education to identify curriculum revisions necessary to prepare students to provide quality care to the frail elderly. None of these goals can be met without a cadre of well-prepared geriatric nursing faculty.

REFERENCES

1. National League for Nursing (1994). *Nursing data review: 1994.* (Pub. No. 19-2639). New York: National League for Nursing.

2. Waters, V., & Sherman, S. *Teaching gerontology.* New York: National League for Nursing Publication #15-241.
3. Johnson, M. A., & Connelly, J. R. (1990). *Nursing and gerontology: Status report.* Washington, DC: Association for Gerontology in Higher Education.
4. Mezey, M., Lynaugh, J., & Cartier, M. (Eds.). (1988*). Aging and academia: The teaching nursing home experience.* New York: Springer Publishing Company.
5. Mezey, M. (1992). Nursing homes: Residents' needs; Nursings' response. In L. Aiken & C. Fagin (Eds.), *Charting Nursing's Future* (pp. 198–215). Philadelphia, PA: Lippincott.
6. Mezey, M., Lynaugh, J., & Cherry, J. (1984). Teaching nursing homes: A report of joint ventures between schools of nursing and nursing homes. *Nursing Outlook, 32,* 136–140.
7. Mezey, M. (1994). Preparation for advanced practice. In M. Mezey & D. McGivern (Eds.*), Nurses, nurse practitioners: Evolution to advanced practice.* New York: Springer Publishing Company.
8. Diers, D., & Molde, S. (1983). Nurses in primary care—The new gatekeepers? *American Journal of Nursing,* 83, 742–745.
9. American Nurses Association (1994). *Accreditation for gerontological practice.* Washington, DC: American Nurses Association.
10. Strumpf, N., Wollman, M. C., & Mezey, M. (1993). Gerontological education for baccalaureate nursing students. *Gerontology & Geriatrics Education, 13,* 3–9.
11. O'Neil, E. H., Leslie, J., Seifer, S., Kahn, J., & Bailiff, P. (Pew Health Professions Commission) (1993). *Nurse practitioners: Doubling the graduates by the year 2000.* Philadelphia: Pew Charitable Trust.
12. Division of Nursing (1994*). Survey of certified nurse practitioners and clinical nurse specialists: December 1992.* (DHHS, Bureau of Health Professions, Health Resources and Services Administration #240-91-0055). Rockville, MD: Author.
13. Strumpf, N., & Paier, G. (1994). Meeting the health care needs of older adults. In M. Mezey & D. McGivern (Eds.), *Nurses, nurse practitioners: Evolution to advanced practice.* New York: Springer Publishing Company.
14. American Nurses Association (1988). *Standards and scope of gerontological nursing practice.* Washington, DC: American Nurses Association.
15. American Nurses Association (1994). *Standards of practice for the primary health care nurse practitioner.* Washington, DC: American Nurses Association.

16. American Nurses Association (1994). *Standards of practice for the clinical specialist.* Washington, DC: American Nurses Association.
17. Mezey, M., Lavizzo-Mourey, R., Brunswick, J., & Taylor, L. (1992). The assessment of nursing home patients. *The Nurse Practitioner, 17,* 50–61.
18. Fulmer, T., & Mezey, M. (1994). Contemporary geriatric nursing. In W. Hazzard, E. Bierman, J. Blass, W. Ettinger, & J. Halter (Eds.), *Principles of geriatric medicine and gerontology* (3rd ed.). New York: McGraw-Hill.
19. Nurse Practitioner and Nurse-Midwifery Program (1993). Rockville, MD: Division of Nursing, DHHS/PHS/HRSA/BHPr.
20. Collings, J. (1986, June 17). *Findings and analysis of ANA practice survey of gerontological nurses.* Presented at the ANA Convention, Anaheim, CA.
21. Ebersole, P. (1985). Gerontological nurse practitioners past and present. *Geriatric Nursing, 6,* 219–22.
22. Buchanan, J., Bell, R., Arnold, S., Wisberger, C., Kane, R., & Garrard, J. (1990, Spring). Assessing cost effects of nursing-home-based geriatric nurse practitioners. *Health Care Financing Review, 11,* 67–78.
23. Kane, R., Garrard, J., Skay, C., Radosevich, D., Buchanan, J., McDermott, S., Arnold, S., & Kepferle, L. (1989). Effect of a geriatric nurse practitioner on the process and outcomes of nursing home care. *American Journal of Public Health, 79,* 1271–77.
24. Garrard, J., Kane, R., Ratner, E., & Buchanan, J. (1990). The impact of nurse clinicians on the care of nursing home residents. In P. Katz, R. Kane, & M. Mezey (Eds.), *Advances in long-term care* (Vol. 1, pp. 169–186). New York: Springer Publishing Company.
25. Annual update of how each state stands on legislative issues affecting advanced nursing practice. (1994). *Nurse Practitioner,* 11–51.
26. Eccard, W. T., & Gainor, E. (1994). Legal ramifications for expanded practice. In M. Mezey & D. McGivern (Eds.), *Nurses, nurse practitioners: Evolution to advanced practice.* New York: Springer Publishing Company.
27. Ebersole, P. (1985). Gerontological nurse practitioners past and present. *Geriatric Nursing, 6,* 219–22.
28. U.S. Congress, Office of Technology Assessment. (1986, December*). Nurse practitioners, physician assistants, and certified nurse-midwives: A policy analysis* (Health Technology Case Study 37, OTA-HCS-37). Washington, DC: U.S. Government Printing Office.
29. Kitzman, H. (1983). The clinical nurse specialist (CNS) and the nurse

practitioner. In A. Hamric & S. Spross (Eds.), *The clinical nurse specialist in theory and practice*. New York: Grune and Stratton.

30. Forbes, K., Rafson, J., Spross, J., & Kozlowski, D. (1990). Clinical nurse specialist and nurse practitioner core curricula survey results. *Nurse Practitioner, 15*, 45–48.

31. Reilly, C. H. (1989). The consultative role of the gerontological nurse specialist in hospitals. *Nursing Clinics of North America, 24*(3), 733–740.

32. Lavizzo-Mourey, R., Mezey, M., & Taylor, L. (1991). Completeness of resident's admission assessments in teaching nursing homes. *Journal of the American Gerontological Society, 39*, 433–439.

33. Minkler, M., Roe, K., & Price, M. (1992). The physical and emotional health of grandmothers raising grandchildren in the crack cocaine epidemic. *The Gerontologist, 32*(6), 752–761.

34. Rubinstein, L. Z., Josephson, K. R., Wieland, G. D., English, P. A., Sayre, J. A., & Kane, R. L. (1984). Effectiveness of a geriatric evaluation unit: A randomized clinical trial. *New England Journal of Medicine, 311*(26), 1664–1670.

35. Siegler, E., & Whitney, F. (1994). Nurse–physician collaboration: Care of adults and the elderly. New York: Springer Publishing Company.

Chapter 2

BARRIERS IN NURSING EDUCATION

Marianne Matzo

U ntil the passage of the Social Security Act in 1935, care of older adults in this country rested primarily with the family or with the state. Organized geriatric nursing began with boarding house care. Elders could not receive both state care and Social Security benefits, so many retired nurses opened their homes to them and provided basic nursing care. Until 1950, geriatric care was the application of general principles of nursing to the aged client, toward the goal of keeping the aged fed, safe, clean, free from pain, and in compliance with the doctors' orders. The study of the aging process, gerontology, did not emerge as a separate discipline until 1960. In 1966, nursing recognized geriatrics as a specialized area of practice (Davis, 1971).

In essence, the nursing profession has had nearly thirty years to integrate gerontological content into nursing education programs, develop innovative clinical experiences for nursing students, and to test this content on national licensing exams. The demographics of the aging population are well known and the multiplicity, chronicity, and duplicity of potential disease processes cannot be disputed. Why, then, is geriatrics not where other specialty areas (e.g., maternal–child health, acute care nursing) are relative to inclusion in the nursing curriculum? Why are there still so few advanced practice nurses who specialize in gerontology? Is there a reason why this is not required content on licensing exams? In 1971, Davis wrote that "only after geriatric nursing is an accepted part of generic programs will we be able to successfully launch and keep graduate programs in geriatric nursing" (p. 11). This chapter will explore why geriatric nursing is still searching for acceptance.

In 1990, the Association for Gerontology in Higher Education (AGHE) published a status report on nursing and gerontology (Johnson & Connelly, 1990). According to the report, many programs rely on growth and development courses to teach gerontological content. The problem with this approach is that growth and development courses tend to focus on the child through young adulthood; when the older adult is mentioned it is usually related to issues of death and dying. This reinforces the perception that the only developmental task facing older persons is to negotiate a good death.

Johnson and Connelly reported further that nursing faculty may presume that because students care for elders in acute or long-term care that this constitutes a gerontological clinical experience. Again, this reinforces a negative stereotype if the only interaction that students have with older persons is with a devitalized population. Advertisers tell us that we "have one chance to make a first impression"; this is also true in gerontological nursing education. If that first view is of a sick or demented older person, then many students may be turned off to this population for the rest of their careers. The lack of an organized plan in the curriculum to introduce students to older adults could have a negative impact on subsequent interactions with older persons.

Ageism (Butler, 1969), the negative view of older persons and the discrimination that accompanies old age, may be another barrier to gerontological content in the nursing curriculum. American society tends to reward those with the greatest economic utility. Some see elders as a drain on society who are willing to take younger workers' tax dollars to fund their Social Security benefits and Medicare health insurance. Nursing faculty may fear their own aging, or fear what they see happening to their own parents and not want to hear about, or teach, age-related changes.

It is surprising that employer mandates have not influenced nursing curricula to a greater extent than they have by demanding that nursing programs educate students about gerontological issues. To cite Johnson and Connelly again, 68% of RNs are employed in acute care, in which 60% of patient days are attributable to older adults. These nurses have had the traditional medical/surgical rotations in their curricula but lack the content relative to what is different about the older adult in these settings.

Since the Johnson and Connelly report was written, there has been an active move toward national health care reform. Currently, most nurses are still employed in acute care, but future trends indicate a move toward community-based and sub-acute care. The NLN's *Nursing's Agenda for Health Care Reform* (1991) is a position statement on how, where, and by whom health care should be delivered; subsequently, the National League for Nursing (NLN) published a *Vision for Nursing Education Reform* (1993). In this report they call for reform so that nursing curricula are more accountable to the public. "Demographics argue for a major focus on care of the elderly and vulnerable populations as well as assurance that education provides a sensitivity and knowledge base that will inform care of diverse cultural and ethnic populations" (NLN, 1993, p. 11).

By the year 2020, 20% of all Americans will be over the age of sixty-five years. The need for gerontological nurses is projected to increase by 466% (ANA, 1986). There are demands in the job market for gerontological nurse practitioners and gero-psychiatric clinical nurse specialists, hospitals are hiring gerontological nurses for their staff development departments, and there is an increased demand for nurse researchers in the area of gerontology. The NLN report cites a national movement "toward greater public accountability for all educational programs," (1993, p. 5), which will result in increased concern for program outcomes and guaranteed competencies of graduates. As educators, we must be forward thinking in curriculum design so that we might meet the public health needs that currently exist and those that will exist in the next century.

These recommendations have yet to become accreditation criteria for which departments of nursing must be accountable. One NLN Criterion states, "The curriculum provides for theoretical and clinical learning activities that focus on clients from diverse populations throughout the life span" (NLN, 1989, p. 7). The realization of this criterion is left open to interpretation by individual schools. If a department of nursing has the faculty with gerontic preparation and/ or interest, then the resulting curriculum can look very different from one where this interest does not exist.

Lack of faculty preparation with a specialty in gerontology has long been cited as a barrier to gerontological content in the nursing curriculum (ANA, 1986; Edel, 1986; Johnson & Connelly, 1990; Mahoney, 1986; Malliarakis & Heine, 1990; Solon, Kilpatrick, & Jill, 1988; Yurchuck & Brower, 1994). Yurchuck and Brower (1994) report that the greatest hindrance to gerontic content inclusion in the nursing curriculum is the lack of faculty members prepared in gerontological nursing. Less than 3% of current faculty members have a masters' degree in gerontological nursing and less than 1% have doctoral preparation in this area (National Institute on Aging, 1987). Yurchuck and Brower's (1994) recent survey of associate and baccalaureate nursing programs in the Southern Regional Education Board (SREB) found that only 12% of faculty members had any preparation in gerontological nursing which was defined as formal preparation, continuing education, or both. Only 5% of both associate and baccalaureate degree faculty had a master's degree with a major or a minor in gerontology. Those with a completed doctoral dissertation in gerontology equaled only 2% of the baccalaureate faculty members and less than half a percent of the associate degree nursing faculty.

Faculty lacking in formal gerontological education continue to hinder the development of gerontological-related content in the nursing curriculum. Yurchik and Brower document that this lack of faculty preparation also impedes clinical experience selection, guidance by clinical role models, generation of excitement for the clinical specialty, and direction of gerontological nursing research. This barrier to gerontological nursing education will continue to exist given that we have yet to see increased numbers of nurses seeking advanced degrees in gerontology. This is not to say, though, that as a discipline we can afford to wait until we have adequate numbers of faculty who can develop this content.

If one of the barriers to gerontological inclusion in the nursing curriculum is the lack of advanced practice nurses, why not focus our attention on recruiting nurses to master's programs in gerontology? Graduate education is built upon the base of generic nursing education (Mahoney, 1986). Gerontological content is irregularly defined and integrated into the associate and baccalaureate degree programs. There are few opportunities for role identification as a gerontic nurse for students at the start of their careers. This shaky foundation does little to support and encourage students to choose gerontology when they decide to pursue a master's degree.

Most departments of nursing are still organized according to the medical model and include curricular content and clinical experiences in the areas of medical/surgical nursing, pediatrics, maternity, and psychology. Given the long history of teaching according to these divisions, many faculty argue that there is not enough time to teach other specialty areas. The changing demographics of this nation support that there are few areas in which nurses practice that they are not primarily providing care to older adults. Johnson and Connelly (1990) take nursing to task when they say that "curricular change has been characterized more by evolution than by revolution," and that "in spite of an identified societal need, nursing faculty often exhibit a cultural lag in responding to calls for change" (p. 5).

There was a time when licensure exams were also organized according to these medical model divisions. This is no longer the case, and the National Council Licensing Examination for Registered Nurses (NCLEX-RN) recruits nurses from all specialty areas to formulate questions for the exam. Content tested on the exam is therefore determined, to some extent, by those who write the questions as well as by the results of the NCLEX-RN validation study.

The purpose of licensure is to guarantee the public that nurses are safe to practice with all age groups. How does the NCLEX-RN exam guarantee to society that the people who pass the exam are truly secure in their knowledge of the older adult? It should be nursing education that responds to the shifting demographics of the country by integrating didactic and clinical experiences with older persons and then requiring that this content be tested on the national licensing exam. If nursing education will not be proactive and change the curriculum on its own, it may be appropriate for the NCLEX-RN to take the lead, test the content, and potentially fail many people taking the exam who have graduated from programs without gerontological content.

It would be unfair to presume that the last thirty years have not resulted in any movement toward integration of gerontological concepts into nursing curricula. Federal funding in the form of Division of Nursing Special Projects Grants have supported departments of nursing in the development of innovative approaches to teaching gerontological nursing. Departments of nursing like those at Saint Anselm College (Matzo, 1993), the University of Pennsylvania (Strumpf, Wollman, & Mezey, 1993), and Old Dominion University (Heine, 1993) have risen to the challenge of rewriting their curricula and integrating gerontological content and clinical experiences. Private foundations, like the W.K. Kellogg Foundation, have funded the Community College-Nursing-Home Partnership, which has also made significant contributions to the development of gerontological content in nursing curricula.

Two years of additional funding were awarded to Saint Anselm College to disseminate what they had learned in the curriculum-revision phase of their grant. Project faculty traveled to baccalaureate and associate-degree programs all over the Northeast to offer insight into the process of gerontological integration. For the most part, we found faculty to be truly interested in how to teach gerontological content and to offer their students what was needed to be informed practitioners when caring for the older adult client.

We also found faculty who had been at their jobs for quite a long time who were teaching what they knew—this content did not include care of the older client. Many of these faculty did not want to have clinical rotations in long-term care, but knew of no other clinical site for gerontological clinical experiences. They were aware of the changing demographics in the United States and felt that the content should be taught, but lacked the motivation to learn a new specialty area and then rewrite lectures to teach that content. Many of the departments of nursing had no new positions to hire faculty with a specialty in gerontology due to budget constraints or the nature of the tenure system, whereby many of the current faculty were at least ten years away from retirement.

We could appreciate their dilemma since we had struggled with some of these issues ourselves. It may well be outside demands, like our accountability to the funding agency, that can be a prime motivator to accomplish the goal of the development of new curricu-

lum models. It may take NLN mandates and gerontological questions on the NCLEX-RN exam to make these changes in a more
generalized fashion in all departments of nursing.

In this chapter, barriers to the integration of gerontology in nursing curricula have been identified. These have included faculty perception of no room for new content in an already full curriculum, ageist
attitudes, the lack of development of gerontological clinical sites, the
lack of prepared faculty to teach the content, the lack of a NLN
mandate for gerontological inclusion in curricula, medical model
underpinnings in nursing curriculum, and the lack of testing of
gerontological content on the NCLEX-RN exam. Davis (1971) ob-
serves that it is only when a group becomes valued for itself and not
for its productive powers that we see progress in the care of members of that group. Twenty-three years ago Davis asked nurses to
"reflect where we came from, view where we are at this moment,
and, hopefully, have a vision of where we are heading" (Davis, 1971,
p. 11). We offer this book as a guide to the actualization of the vision
of thoughtful and inclusive gerontological content in nursing curricula,
meaningful clinical experiences with a wide variety of older adults in
varied settings, significant and scholarly nursing research relative
to the older adult, and enough dedicated advance practice nurses
to continue this vision into the next millennium.

REFERENCES

American Nurses Association. (1986). *Gerontological nursing curriculum.*
Kansas City, MO: Author.
Butler, R. (1969). Age-ism: Another form of bigotry. *Gerontologist, 9,* 243.
Davis, B. A. (1971, Winter). Geriatric nursing through the looking glass. *The
Journal of the New York State Nurses Association,* 7–12.
Edel, M. K. (1986). Recognize gerontological Content. *Journal of Geronto-
logical Nursing, 12*(10), 28–32.
Heine, C. (ed.). (1993). *Determining the future of gerontological nursing
education: Partnerships between education and practice.* NY: NLN
Press.
Johnson, M. A., & Connelly, J. R. (1990). *Nursing and gerontology: Status
report.* Washington, DC: Association for Gerontology in Higher Education.

Mahoney, D. F. (1986). Gerontological nursing in graduate education. In E. C. Gioiella (Ed.), *Gerontology in the professional nursing curriculum* (pp. 63–86). New York: NLN Pub. No. 15–2151.

Malliarakis, D. R., & Heine, C. (1990). Is Gerontological nursing included in baccalaureate nursing programs? *Journal of Gerontological Nursing, 16*(6), 4–7.

Matzo, M. (ed.). (1993). Integrating Gerontology into the Nursing Curriculum. *Gerontology and Geriatrics Education, 13*(3), 3–106.

National Institute on Aging. (1987). *Personnel for health needs of the elderly through 2020.* Washington DC: U.S. Department of Health and Human Services.

National League for Nursing. (1991). *Nursing's agenda for Health Care Reform.* New York: NLN Press.

National League for Nursing. (1993). *A vision for nursing education.* New York: NLN Press.

National League for Nursing, Council of Baccalaureate and Higher Degree Programs. (1989). *Criteria for the Evaluation of Baccalaureate and Higher Degree Programs in Nursing* (pp. 15–1251). New York: Author.

Oasis. (1986). Staff. American Nurses Association, 8, 4.

Solon J. A., Kilpatrick, N. S., & Jill, M. S. (1988). Aging related education: A national survey. *Journal of Gerontological Nursing, 14*(9), 21–26.

Strumpf, N. E., Wollman, M. C., & Mezey, M. D. (1993). Gerontological education for Baccalaureate nursing students. *Gerontology and Geriatrics Education, 13*(3), 73–84.

Yurchuck, E. R, & Brower, H. T. (1994, January). Faculty preparation for gerontological nursing. *Journal of Gerontological Nursing,* 17–24.

Chapter 3

Incorporating Geriatrics into the Licensure and Accreditation Process

Terry Fulmer and Mary Tellis Nyack

W hile faculty with keen interests in geriatric nursing continue to teach their elective courses, nothing will move gerontological nursing firmly into the curriculum until licensing and monitoring by professional educational accrediting bodies mandate such content. The process begins with valuing: all documents by prestigious American nursing organizations such as the American Nurses Association (ANA), the National League for Nursing (NLN), and the American Academy of Nursing (AAN), for example, must speak out on the value of gerontological nursing content and follow it by recognizing the need for required content.

The ANA has provided certification in gerontological nursing since the late 70s, and there is now a move to have gerontological nursing certification at the master's level, as is the case with other specialties. This is an important signal that gerontological nursing is of equal status and value as other specialties. Specific organizational certification has not yet happened, but will likely become a point of discussion in the next decade.

Licensing for registered nurses cannot take place without sitting for board certification. To date, there are few questions related to

29

specific gerontological nursing content, and until those areas are developed, neither students nor faculty will see any reason to provide adequate curricular content in this area. Areas such as normal aging and its sequelae, functional status in the elderly, pharmaco-therapeutics with regard to elders, and specialty sections on common problems in the elderly such as incontinence, pressure sores, confusion management, restraints and their sequelae, and falls, are all critical to appropriate nursing care of the elderly. Additional topics such as healthy aging and health promotion as it affects the elderly are also essential. Without appropriate examination of these topics, there is little incentive to provide curricular content and to encourage mastery of such knowledge. Leaders in the field should volunteer to be item writers for the gerontological nursing questions that should be included in standardized exams. These same leaders would analyze examinations for gerontological content and develop an evaluation blueprint to encourage a proactive stance on this topic. Analysis should determine the current percentage of gerontological exam content and yield a target percentage for the future. Since reimbursement is tied to geriatric nurse practitioner certification, it is important to lobby for this content at the graduate level and for at least some exposure during advance practice nursing adult studies.

Nursing assistant certification was mandated under OBRA in 1987. To build upon this important step, appropriate monies should be allocated for mentoring these individuals for the continuum of education they might pursue. Nursing assistants might consider becoming a licensed practical nurse, a registered nurse in an associate degree program, or a registered nurse in a baccalaureate program. The major disparity in health care between acute-care salaries and nursing-home salaries must also be addressed.

Many nursing facilities are entering into the arena of subacute care. Facilities (units) offering subacute care will help nurses move from acute to long-term care; it may also provide opportunities for gerontological nursing in a setting more familiar to the acute-care experienced nurse. Nurses working in subacute care must also be educated to respect the expertise of the LTC nurse who has extensive experience with the regulation necessary to remain licensed.

The NLN's accreditation process for curriculum also needs to be revised. The current NLN language, which speaks to providing content across the life-span, must be made more specific with regard to describing mandated gerontological nursing curriculum content. Without licensing and NLN accreditation to change the gerontological nursing curriculum content, its content will continue to be by whim and the influence of "interested" faculty. It is well known that as faculty with interest in gerontological nursing change positions, the content may well be lost. A three-credit course should be mandated in every undergraduate program, with accompanying required clinical experience. Such a mandate would send a strong message to students that geriatric content is valued and acknowledged, and that the school is keeping up with society in global demographic trends. Some might say that such a mandate would usurp the autonomy of the faculty with regard to curriculum development. The same could be said for pediatrics, obstetrics, and psychiatric nursing, but to date these areas are not perceived as problematic.

Finally, an extremely effective way to disseminate research findings to practicing nurses is to incorporate new knowledge into testing mechanisms. It may be two to three years before a textbook is available to the public from the time of its inception. Incorporating new research findings in the examination for licensing process can enhance the communication of new findings. Table 3.1 lists current research programs related to aging and nursing, funded by NIH.

A national mandate through the NLN should ensure that gerontological nursing content is taught. Regulation without caution can be troublesome to faculty and students alike, but to date we have spent 20 years discussing gerontological content and very little has occurred. There has been no systematic study of gerontological content in the curriculum since Brower's 1979 survey. A new survey is absolutely essential to ensure that appropriate elderly citizens, whose ranks are increasing dramatically, are receiving nursing care.

There is a need to evaluate the effect of curriculum on nursing practice with a clinical-based outcome measurement in testing. There is also a need for competency examinations that identify key outcomes and build upon the ANA standards for gerontological nursing (ANA, 1987) at the basic and advanced level. Currently, the NLN has divided competencies among AD, BS, and graduate programs,

TABLE 3.1   NIH Research Programs in Nursing and Aging 1987–1992

Investigator	Project Title	Project #
Lois K. Evans University of Pennsylvania	Reducing Restraints in Nursing Homes—A Clinical Trial	5R01AGO8324-03
Barbara K. Haight Medical University of South Carolina	Life Review—Prevention of Depression and Suicidality (Human)	5R29MH45323-03
Nancy I. Bergstrom University of Nebraska Medical Center	Nursing Assessment of Pressures or Risks (Human)	5R01NR01061-06
Virginia K. Neelon University of North Carolina	Acute Confusion in Hospitalized Elderly—Patterns and Factors	5RO1NR01339-07
Nancy E. Reame University of Michigan	Nursing Assessment—Menstrual Cycle Clinical Models	5R01NR01373-06
Thelma J. Wells University of Rochester	Nursing Interventions—Exercise for Stress Incontinence	5RO1NRO1917-05
Patricia A. Gillett University of Utah	Nurse Exercise Intervention for Overweight Older Women	5R29NRO2087-03
Patricia G. Archbold Oregon Health Science University	Evaluation of Care Giving Support Program	5RO1NRO2088-02
Mary D. Naylor University of Pennsylvania	Comprehensive Discharge Planning for the Elderly	2RO1NRO2095-04
Margaret J. Bull University of Minnesota	Testing a Model for Hospital To Home Transition	5RO1NRO2249-02
Sally P. Weinrich University of South Carolina	Nursing Interventions To Increase Colorectal Screening in the Elderly	3RO1NRO2259-02S1
Cornelia M. Beck University of Arkansas	Improving Dressing Behavior in Impaired Elderly	5RO1NRO2367-03
Barbara J. Bowers University of Wisconsin	Caregiver Perceptions of Caring For Older Adults	5RO1NRO2405-02
Mary B. Engler University of California at San Francisco	Omega-3 Fatty Acids and Cardiovascular Risk Factors	1R29NRO2407-01A2
Beverly L. Roberts Case Western Reserve University	Walking—A Nursing Intervention	5RO1NRO2575-02
Sharol Jacobson University of Oklahoma	Diabetic Representations and Signs of Mvskoke Indians	5RO1NRO2618-02
Jana M. Mossey Medical College of Pennsylvania	Nurse Intervention With Depressed Medically Ill Elderly	5RO1NRO2642-02
Muriel B. Ryden University of Minnesota	Treating Aggression Through Dementia Care Education	5RO1NRO2965-02
Suzanne R. Van Ort University of Arizona	Nursing Interventions for Preserving Meal time Behaviors	1RO1NRO3034-01

TABLE 3.1 (*continued*)

Investigator	Project Title	Project #
Carole A. Mitchell Montefiore Medical Center	Management of Resistance to Bathing Activities	5RO1AG10644-02
Molly C. Dougherty University of Florida at Gainesville	Circumvaginal Muscle Function— Clinical Interventions	5RO1NRO1115-07
Linda R. Phillips University of Arizona	Cultural and Causal Factors in the Quality of Family Caregiving	5RO1NRO1323-07
Joan K. Magilvy University of Colorado Health Sciences Center	Rural Home Care for Older Adults—Patterns and Process	5RO1NRO2006-03
Marquis D. Foreman University of Illinois at Chicago	Confusion—A Three Wave Longitudinal Causal Model	5R29NR02231-02
Beatrice J. McDowell University of Pittsburgh	Behavior Treatment of Incontinence in Homebound Elderly	1R01NRO2874-01A1
Jean F. Wyman Medical College of Virginia	Urinary Incontinence in Community Dwelling Women	5U01AGO5170-08
Andrea M. Barsevick Fox Chase Career Center	Factors Affecting Recovery From Hip Surgery	5R29NRO1839-06
Mary P. Quayhagen University of San Diego	Cognitive Stimulation Training in Alzheimer Families	5RO1NRO1931-03

but the publication lacks distinctions: more needs to be done in this realm.

Monitoring by the NLN with regard to gerontological nursing content provides an opportunity for on-site visits that ensure such content is being delivered. However, since the NLN monitors only the synthesis of curriculum, the only way to do it is to make it an NLN criterion. The NLN should be encouraged to have a sub-group on gerontological nursing within its councils. Faculty need to support curricular resolutions based on data from research studies, which outline why such content is needed. The State Board Test Pool can be influenced by community pressure, composition of membership, and emphasis of that board. Minimum requirements for gerontological content within the state board test pool should be determined. It should not be construed that this chapter advocates for a question based on age alone. The need for expert mastery must be based on knowledge of clinical presentations in the elderly and outcomes of specific interventions. Further, more information about the cohorts and their differences (ages 65–74; 75–84, etc.) must be added and tested.

Mandating continuing education for those practicing with aging individuals is another way to ensure high-quality practice with the elderly. More emphasis should be placed on the value of long-term nursing, including mandated long-term care content within the undergraduate curriculum, and certainly within the graduate area of gerontological nursing. Students need to understand how they will be responsible for the management of nursing assistants, the delegation of work activities, and working with state surveyors who come to evaluate practice. Proactive planning now will enable more influential people to become interested and a certain public saturation to occur. In our era of health care reform, which emphasizes high quality cost effectiveness and documentation of outcomes, there is an opportunity to make a strong case for gerontological nursing. Stabilized funding is needed for gerontological care, and the argument needs to be made based on health-services research that looks at the quality of life and health promotion with regard to excellence in gerontological nursing. Until the requisite data can be gathered to show changes, we will continue to be challenged on the value of specific content in our field.

We must use our approval and licensing procedures to motivate those who direct curriculum to include gerontological nursing. In addition, we need to recognize and support creative initiatives, perhaps through a better model for gerontological nursing or through using the Freis model of rectangularization with maintenance of maximum function of goal throughout the lifespan. Finally, we need to use our political organizations to influence administrators, funding sources, scholarship sources, and federal research initiatives for this important endeavor. Regulations need to reflect the needs and demands of the American public without discrimination by age.

The consequences of failing to make these changes include intergenerational warfare where young and old continue to be pitted against each other with regard to curriculum and funding, higher costs in terms of poor nursing care of incontinence, restraints, over-medication of the elderly, and polypharmacy; and data need to be generated to describe the costs in terms of morbidity and mortality. Such data might be obtained from the Hospital Outcomes Project for the Elderly, funded by the John A. Hartford Foundation of New York City, which lays out costs of functional decline in hospitalized elderly. Further, the MacArthur Foundation, the Baltimore Longitudinal Aging Study, and the National Institute on Aging data should further the argument for gerontological nursing content.

REFERENCES

American Nurses Association. (1987). *Standards and scope of gerontological nursing practice.* Kansas City, MO: Author.
National League for Nursing. (1993). *NLN accreditation standards.* New York: NLN.

Chapter 4

Expanding Clinical Experiences

May L. Wykle and Carol M. Musil

As nursing educators grapple with decisions about incorporating gerontological nursing content and clinical experiences into their curricula, it is worthwhile to consider that by the next century, those age 65 will likely live another 20 years. By comparison, the pediatric years are 18 years at most, and maternity care—from pre-conception counseling to the six-week check-up, even if a woman has several maternity cycles—reaches only a fraction of the geriatric years. Just as the childbearing years and the pediatric years are times of enormous development and change for the individual and family, the years from 65 to 85 also hold many changes that are equally remarkable in their pervasiveness, and profoundly transform the lives of individuals and families.

Many nursing educational programs provide opportunities early in the student's career to follow a family, generally during the childbearing year, for exposure to family, child and adult development, for continuity of care, and to assess maternal-child health needs in various settings. Occasionally, nursing and medical school programs have teamed students in pairs to learn initial collaborative skills while together following an "expanding family." An additional contemporary clinical experience would be to link health-professions students with the young-old, middle-old, or old-old, who will show a variety of developmental changes associated with aging over the course of the four years of nursing and medical school.

This chapter will examine the many issues and concerns about developing clinical sites and expanding the range of geriatric clinical opportunities available to graduate and undergraduate nursing students. Expectations of students and new resources for gerontological nursing placements will be considered.

ISSUES AND CONCERNS

Two of the greatest barriers faced by gerontologists are overcoming the limited perspective that society has toward aging and debunking the illness myths that surround aged persons. These negative images of aging are gradually, albeit slowly, shifting. With each cohort of elders, the absolute numbers of older adults who are sicker may increase, but proportionately more older adults, especially those under age 75, will enjoy better physical and mental health for a longer period of time (Cohen, 1992). These well elders are not often available to students through the channels most frequently used to access patients, for example, hospitals and nursing homes. Other valuable sources that would provide students an opportunity to interact with well elders outside the health-care system exist, and new relationships and approaches must be developed to access them. For example, students can provide services that bring them in contact with community-dwelling elders, or they could accompany well elders in their various activities. Meeting the needs of students while responding to changes in the health-care system and community expectations offers many possibilities for gerontic clinical sites that have not yet been fully realized.

Generic Student Issues

Another problem is how to recruit students into gerontological nursing. New nursing graduates do not select gerontological nursing for their clinical education even though most nurses will encounter geriatric patients in their practice. Enhancing the prestige of nursing the aged is a challenge, although changes in the health-care system as well as in the aging of those receiving the largest share of health care ought to modify this perspective. Self-reliance and independence are critical attributes for nurses working with elderly persons in long-term care, whether it is in the community or in institutionalized settings. Selecting nursing homes as a first clinical experience can impede the goal of enhancing the image of gerontological nursing since beginning students are often insecure working with frail elders. Early in their baccalaureate careers, nursing students are prepared to evaluate patients' needs at a basic level and focus on physical care. Older adults need psychosocial care as well, and their person–environment interactions may be more complicated. Without an opportunity to revisit the health-care needs of older adults at a later stage in their educational preparation, students may underestimate the complexity of planning care for older adults. Thus, rather than recognizing how health and capability are balanced with decreasing physiologic resilience in elderly adults, some students will conceptualize geriatric nursing as no more than skills and tasks to be performed on the old or infirm.

Faculty and Curriculum Issues

In part, negative perceptions of aging stem from faculty images and expectations about care of the "older patient." Although all conceptual models of nursing ascribe a central focus to health, even for individuals approaching death, articulating and implementing this direction has been troublesome with the older adult population. Finding time in the curriculum to add holistic content on aging and to plan relevant clinical experiences requires renegotiation of other content and rethinking about the expected outcomes of nursing education. Combined with the tasks of attending to the developmental needs of students, the placement of gerontological nursing in the baccalaureate curriculum requires careful consideration. Inspiring students to initiate care for older patients is not an easy task. Students often view care of the aged as chronic, dull, and routine. A range of opportunities for eldercare do exist, and many may enhance the image of caring for the older adult while helping students to develop professional skills (Wykle & Kaufman, 1988).

Many new nurses are minimally competent to work with older adults after graduating from a basic program even when they have had well-planned integrated class content in the care of the elderly adult. Theory-based clinical practice is needed for them to achieve the judgment and individual performance desired. Students need two types of experiences, giving care and coordinating care, which may be acquired at different stages of educational preparation. For example, a beginning focus on communication with older adults enhances the student's ability to work in a variety of settings where elders are found. Preceptorships and independent studies are also two viable options to increase the opportunities available to students to develop expertise in the care of elders. Another possibility is to offer internships after graduation that would give the new graduate more clinical experience with the aged. In times of a tight job market, such clinical exposure provides a chance for nurses to improve clinical skills upon entering the health-care system.

In addition to clinical skills, generic students need basic skills practice in management, delegation, and accountability to support the advanced roles of team leaders and case managers that they will eventually assume. Concurrently, there must be role clarity and parity across specialties. That is, clear definitions and expectations of roles for team member, case manager, team leader, and advanced practice are necessary to lend validity to all roles, regardless of specialty, but particularly in long-term care where these skills are essential. In sum, we need a gerontological nursing model that incorporates health promotion, systems thinking, care management, a developmental human life-cycle approach, and adequate clinical experience.

ALTERNATIVE CLINICAL SITES

Opportunities to capture the continuity of care across the geriatric years are available in the community, in acute- and long-term care, and in home health care. In addition, a number of new possibilities for clinical placements can be developed.

Generic Students

Baccalaureate nurses need a gradient of experiences based on life-span development of individuals. Planning the curriculum to in-

clude relevant theory and alternative clinical experiences in gerontology will require coordination with other clinical rotations.

Community Nursing

There are untapped opportunities for clinical experiences with the
young-, middle- and oldest-old in the community. Further, the community may have a variety of organizations, such as "senior citizen"
organizations and "golden-age" centers, where students may observe and interact with well elderly clients. Development of these
settings as viable clinical sites is most likely to occur when needs of
families in the community drive the clinical services provided. For
example, clinics in housing and shopping centers might be used as
clinical sites for more advanced students. Clinical objectives planned
with the community and tailored to fit a given site or focus, such as
day care, hi-rise living, senior centers, or nutrition sites can create
valuable learning experiences while building important bridges with
the community. There remains a strong need to develop ethnic sites
where culturally sensitive geriatric nursing care can be delivered,
particularly to African-American, Latino, and Asian-American elders
(Wykle & Kaskel, 1991).

Some community health centers and demonstration projects
such as OnLok and Pace that provide continuity of care for older
adults are prototypical clinical placements. Using well elderly visi-
tors to the classroom might be another opportunity to expand perspectives on aging. These well elderly who have not been identified
within the health-care system provide a view of the life-span development that is often not recognized. These individuals who can be
teachers of the young can be contacted through churches and community senior groups.

Opportunities can also be provided for some students to learn more
about home care for elderly individuals who have not been referred
through the typical health-care network. Such individuals may have
had referrals from their pastors or from the local office on aging. In
rural communities, referral models such as these have provided excellent clinical opportunities, although faculty resources and logistics
are sometimes constraining. Managing the supervision of undergraduate nursing students in various well-elder sites is time-consuming and

not always practical for one person. Since generic students require close faculty supervision, approximately one faculty member per eight students, this limitation should be acknowledged as a challenge so that planning for adequate supervision can occur.

Acute Care

The majority of patients in acute-care hospitals and hospital clinics are over 65. Students may have a specific older adult experience once they have had gerontological theory. Acute-care settings provide many role models, including clinical managers, clinical nurse specialists, and nurse practitioners, and offer the opportunity to work with interdisciplinary teams, such as geriatric-assessment teams.

Long-Term Care

Although some of the limitations of clinical placements in nursing homes have already been discussed, working with elders in such environments gives students a nonstressful experience with appreciative clients. Following older adults from an acute, transitional, skilled facility back to home affords the sense of progress, healing, and adaptation that can be gained when taking a longitudinal rather than cross-sectional view. Students need both integrated and specialized experiences. Clinical experiences with older adults that integrate clinical knowledge include hospices, continuing-care retirement centers, and intergenerational day-care sites. Community mental health centers are also potential locations for geriatric nursing care.

Home Health Care

Home health care, whether for short-term or long-term support of patients and their families, is the wave of the future. Clinical experiences with home health agencies or visiting nurse associations are critical components of an undergraduate curriculum, especially in relation to the care of elders, where 80 percent of those needing care are at home in the community.

Other Options

Another emerging possibility is a faculty gerontological nursing practice that includes geriatric case managers and clinical nurse specialists in elder care, long-term care, and community health. In these practices, students can work with faculty to develop appropriate clinical skills and learn to function *inter*dependently. Nursing home-community college partnerships provide a real opportunity for making a constructive impact on the health of elders in the local community. An innovative but pertinent clinical experience is to pair students with caregiving families for a semester. In nursing programs where case management is a focus throughout clinical training, students begin to take the long, rather than short view, of patient and family experiences with health states.

Graduate Clinical Training Sites

A geriatric nursing case manager can be expected to coordinate a high level of skilled physical and psychosocial care. Geriatric nurse practitioner students can begin with health promotion and wellness in an appropriate site. Ambulatory sites with other nurse practitioners are excellent resources, particularly if a master's-prepared nurse practitioner is on site to serve as a preceptor. Graduate students may also track patients through various settings of managed care, acute care, and in the community. Having the opportunity to work in a collaborative practice setting in graduate school will complement the theoretical component of master's education and provide the student a reality-based ideal. This offering of longitudinal experiences becomes essential. The use of case studies can be a preparatory experience to convey how the long-term nurse–client relationship might unfold.

To increase the number of nurse practitioners prepared to meet the needs of older adults, all adult nurse practitioner programs should include a strong gerontology clinical training component, in addition to the education of geriatric nurse practitioners and clinical specialists. Geriatric clinical specialist students require exposure to acute- and long-term care, both in nursing homes and in the community. Supervision of home health aides and licensed practical nurses is also an important component of the clinical management experience at the graduate level. Developing consultation skills in the care of elderly persons is a necessary aspect of graduate education.

MENTAL HEALTH CLINICAL EXPERIENCES

Given the prevalence of psychiatric symptoms and cognitive impairment among older adults, nursing students need guided academic experiences to work with older adult psychiatric patients, either in adult, psychiatric, or community-health settings. Essential experiences include interviewing, psychosocial and functional assessments, and counseling family and support persons. The use of nursing homes as a learning site depends upon availability and the resources on premises. Individual and particularly group therapy with older adults in nursing homes has been quite successful (Abraham, Niles, Theil, Siarkowski, & Cowling, 1991). Interactive computer-based learning packages and modules need to be developed not only for students but also for use by faculty who may be less prepared to teach geropsychiatric content.

Graduate Students

Graduate students in gerontology and mental-health nursing may be most prepared to address psychiatric and psychosocial issues of nursing home patients. These students can attend, conduct, and analyze geriatric therapy groups, including reminiscence, remotivation, and psychotherapy groups. Again, individual counseling and guided imagery are useful to nursing home residents. Hospitals with acute-care geriatric units may also be a place where graduate students might organize short-term groups. Even if the groups are small and individuals can attend only one or two sessions, the group members dealing with existential issues often create powerful therapeutic encounters for themselves and their caregivers. Opportunities for consultation and to conduct individual or family therapy and crisis groups with nursing home residents are available if staff know that graduate nursing students are resources for these services. Psychosocial home-care interventions, including assessment, home teaching, and psychosocial support to informal caregivers, provided through visiting nurse and home-care agencies, are critical learning experiences that will form the bulk of future nursing practice.

Undergraduate Students

Nursing homes may be ideal locations for developing initial psycho-social skills and examining communication issues. Cognitively intact elders are often very articulate and willing to share their experiences and insights with students. Process recordings with geriatric patients are quite useful for helping students to review basic communication techniques and for exploring themes related to health, life-span development, loss, and functional dependence. While the mental health content of gerontology is essential to understanding of the older adult, psychopathology and mental illnesses associated with aging are also requisite knowledge. Theory about crisis intervention, assessment and referral of elders, introductory knowledge about the relationship between cognitive, psychological, and physiological functioning in elderly adults, and the use of psychoactive medications by elderly adults are essential content for undergraduate gerontological clinical experiences.

FACULTY REQUIREMENTS

Currently, there is more emphasis from regulatory bodies, for example, state boards of nursing, to incorporate gerontological nursing into the curriculum. In addition to theory for both gerontology and geriatric mental health nursing, clinical experience is a critical part of the curriculum. Whether these changes are mandated or chosen, their timely success depends on having appropriate faculty resources. Without a faculty role model or geriatric advocate, the movement to incorporate a life-span developmental approach (Reed, 1983) will be impeded. Developing knowledge among faculty about older adults, especially the oldest-old, is essential. A first step is for faculty to examine their own assumptions about the physical and mental health of the elderly. For example, the issue of suicide among older adults or the very ill raises many ethical questions that are to be considered. Further, sensitivity to students' developmental learning needs about aging is an essential part of curriculum planning. Preparatory to clinical work, students require systems and critical thinking skills. Additionally, the curriculum could have appropriate support courses from the behavioral sciences and humanities to undergird this broader base of gerontic knowledge.

Although the problems of time and faculty resources exist, by identifying a core set of skills and clinical experiences, the expectations for student learning can be explicated and then shared. As the number of geriatric nursing faculty prepared at the doctoral and postdoctoral level increases, the ways in which relevant content is developed and integrated into the curriculum will also increase. To extend the base of academic clinical support, master's and doctoral students can be used to supervise beginning students in agencies. Experiences in which new students shadow older students provide a "learning-by-watching" model, but also afford early mentorship experiences for older students. This model has been successfully used by the medical discipline for years to inculcate values, behaviors, and skills to students learning the profession. Along with supervision through teamwork, having students work with more advanced students, or even utilizing qualified professionals from other disciplines who qualify for clinical faculty appointments, increases the number of available student options. Another means of expanding the geriatric faculty base would be to have qualified directors of nursing in nursing homes serve as mentors of gerontological nursing students (Wykle & Kaufman, 1988).

In sum, there is an urgent need to provide a range of geriatric clinical opportunities to nursing students at all levels if we are to meet the health-care challenges of the next century and the dramatic increase in frail elders. Success, however, depends on the faculty believing in the significance of the life-span developmental framework for nursing (Reed, 1983) and in the value of gerontological clinical experiences for nursing students.

REFERENCES

Abraham, I., Niles, S., Theil, B., Siarkowski, K., & Cowling, R. (1991). Therapeutic group work with depressed elderly. *Nursing Clinics of North America, 23*(3), 635–650.

Cohen, G. (1992). The future of mental health and aging. In J. Birren, R. B. Sloane, & G. Cohen, (Eds.), *Handbook of mental health and aging* (2nd ed., pp. 893–914). San Diego, CA: Academic Press, Inc.

Reed, P. (1983). Implications of the life-span developmental framework for well-being in adulthood and aging. *Advances in Nursing Science, 6*, 18–25.

Wykle, M., & Kaskel, B. (1991). Increasing the longevity of minority older adults through improved health status. In *Minority elders: Longevity, economics, and health-building a public policy base* (pp. 24–31). Washington, DC, Special Issue of Gerontological Society of America.

Wykle, M., & Kaufman, M. (1988). The teaching nursing home experiences—Case Western Reserve (OH)/Margaret Wagner House. In M. B. Walsh & N. R. Small (Eds.), *Teaching nursing homes: The nursing perspective*. Rockville, MD: National Health Publishing.

Chapter 5

Student Resistance:
Overcoming Ageism

Carla Mariano

Ageism has been defined as a "tendency to impose limitations or expectations related solely to chronological age" (Ebersole & Hess, 1990, p. 833). Robert Butler (1975) described ageism as "a process of systematic stereotyping of and discrimination against people because they are old . . . Ageism allows the younger generations to see older people as different from themselves; thus they subtly cease to identify with their elders as human beings" (p. 12). These stereotypes and biases employed to define older persons exclusively because of their age are "an attempt by younger generations to shield themselves from the fact of their own eventual aging and death and to avoid having to deal with the social and economic problems of increasing numbers of older people" (Butler, Lewis, & Sunderland, 1991, p. 176).

At the 1994 conference, "Caring for older Americans: The critical role of nursing education," the preconceptions and prejudices that create and perpetuate student resistance to caring for the elderly were identified. Also discussed were proposed solutions to overcoming ageism among nursing students. This chapter summarizes the thinking of the participants and discusses the outcomes of those discussions in the context of related literature.

PSYCHOLOGICAL/EMOTIVE BARRIERS

One of the major contributors to student ageism is the fear that is associated with aging, often directly related to myths and strongly held beliefs about this population. Matteson and McConnell (1988) [citing Solomon, 1982] note that common stereotypes regard older people as "dependent, asexual, pessimistic toward the future, insecure, meddlesome, lonely, not valued by their families, and in poor physical and mental condition and have memory loss and limited interests" (p. 483). Eyde and Rich (1983) suggest that three of the most damaging stereotypes are that aging means homogeneity, that is, the elderly lose their individuality and become more alike; aging means senility; and aging results in rigidity, inflexibility, and contrariness or "crotchety and complaining." Butler (1969) says further, "Ageism reflects a deep-seated uneasiness . . . a personal revulsion to and distaste for growing old, disease, disability and fear of powerlessness, 'uselessness' and death" (p. 245).

With these not-uncommon social attitudes, values, and beliefs about older people, it is no wonder that students are often turned off to working with the elderly. It is also not surprising that they (and oftentimes faculty), through projection of their future selves, dread the reality of their own aging and thereby deny consideration of it by avoiding learning about aging or dealing with the elderly.

Other forms of ageism may be equally discriminating and destructive. Kalish (1979) has described a "new ageism" where the elderly are stereotyped by care providers as being the least capable, least healthy, and least alert, as well as helpless, dependent, and dysfunctional without the assistance of health and social agencies and organizations. Services are developed or mandated regardless of the potential for decreasing the freedom of the older person to make his or her own decisions. This conception can produce dependency and helplessness in elderly clients. Kalish proposes that the "new ageism" is based on failure models. These models imply that the elderly person is incompetent and will inevitably "fail," if not now then in the future. These models further convey to the elderly that they are powerless to deal with their own aging and societal victimization without professional assistance. As Burnside and Schmidt

(1994) note, "Some capable older people have been undermined by ageism; they accept dependency roles that deny them leadership roles" (p. 92).

There are a number of activities that can combat the denial, fear, and psychological/emotive barriers to student interest in caring for the elderly. The above describes negative attitudes about aging. Students must be introduced to more positive and optimistic views of aging. Ebersole and Hess (1990), in their book, *Toward Healthy Aging,* discuss other perspectives on aging. Some of these include "Aging as Living," "Aging as Education," "Aging as Art," "Aging as a Spiritual Journey," and "Aging as a Peak Experience." Viewed from Martha Rogers's framework, aging is negentropic or characterized by "increasing heterogeneity, differentiation, diversity, and complexity" (Barrett, 1990). As Rogers (1986) states, "Aging is not a disease. . . . Contrary to a static view engendered by a closed-system model of the universe which postulates aging to be a running down, the Science of Unitary Human Beings postulates aging to be a developmental process. Aging is continuous, from conception through dying. Field patterns are increasingly diverse and creative . . . Innovative developmental diversity manifests itself nonlinearly . . . More diverse field patterns change more rapidly than the less diverse" (p. 7). Recasting the image of the elderly in an affirmative light facilitates not only the conception but also the attitudes of students regarding elderly persons.

Students need to learn about successful aging as well as atypical biopsychosocial changes in functional capabilities. Stereotypic images need to be contrasted with factual information about both healthy and ill older persons. Presenting the nursing role in rehabilitation care and recovery can foster a more realistic picture of the strengths as well as problems of the elderly. Increased exposure to all aspects of gerontology, especially well-elder experiences, will demonstrate to students the diversity of the older population. This also will provide the opportunity for nursing students to witness firsthand the vitality, potential, abilities, and healthy aging of elderly people. Use of poetry, letters, and films, as well as helping students develop and maintain a relationship with an older person over time cultivates in the student both understanding and empathy toward the elderly (Matzo, 1993).

Insight workshops, conducted as part of the educational program, help students to understand and directly confront the phenomenon of aging and explore their own feelings, values, attitudes, and beliefs related to growing older. Tiemann and Stone (1990) offer some exceedingly useful experiential teaching techniques for assisting students to gain insight into, reflect upon, and anticipate the processes of aging. Additionally, students should be encouraged to engage in candid but supportive discussions of coping, grief, death, bereavement, and reminiscence.

Faculty themselves may also unwittingly model ageist conceptions and behaviors. Comparison of one's own occasional forgetful behavior with Alzheimer's may have unintended consequences on students solidifying the stereotype that the aged are demented. Aversion to the elderly on the part of faculty may well be related to negative stereotypes of nursing students toward the elderly. O'Reilly and Kazanowski (1993) suggest that nursing faculty assess their own attitudes toward older persons using a tool such as the Cook and Pieper questionnaire (Cook & Pieper, 1985). It is also helpful for faculty as a whole to discuss how stereotypical viewpoints slip into discourse about the elderly and the need to avoid ageism in the teaching/learning process.

Students often have the preconception that all gerontology takes place in nursing homes with demented and sick aged people. In a study of the impact of attitudes in care of the aged, Nay-Brock (1988) found that the first words student nurses associated with old age included euthanasia, wrinkled, slow, lonely, in the way, frail, cranky, false teeth, throw-away, wise, decrepit, walking stick, and kind. Again, students need broad exposure to a variety of settings in which older people reside. It is crucial that nursing students see the variety and diversity of this population on the entire health continuum. Students should be encouraged to tell their own stories, both positive and negative, about their dealings with older people. Faculty should also use the technique of storytelling to weed out biases about the elderly and to capture the richness of older persons' lives. The importance of "stereotype testing"—giving factual information on aging, for example, 67 percent of older, noninstitutionalized people live in a family setting with a spouse, relative, or friend, and 76 percent live in their own homes (Aging America, 1991)—cannot be underestimated when combating ageism.

However, there is the reality that approximately five percent of those over the age of 65 are in nursing homes at any one time, and one in five elderly persons will spend some time in a nursing home during their remaining years (Aging America, 1991; Mezey, 1994). Learning to provide nursing care for those in long-term care facilities and nursing homes must be a part of the experience for nursing students. Students need content on and skill in dealing with the physical, psychological, and ethical aspects of chronic illness. Dementia, delirium, and depression are common manifestations about which students express much apprehension. With proper teaching and supportive practice experiences, students can successfully care for elderly persons with these symptoms.

Lastly, students themselves need the ability to cope. "Care for the caretaker" is a concept of immeasurable importance when managing elderly patients with chronic physical, emotional, and cognitive disorders. When students are taught stress management strategies (such as simple relaxation, meditation, guided imagery, and cognitive restructuring techniques), in addition to appropriate care practices, they are helped to develop empathic resilience. What might have been perceived as a potentially negative and overwhelming event will be handled with greater mastery, thereby instilling feelings of competence and confidence in the student. A student's self-image of proficiency and accomplishment when caring for the elderly can itself counter negative and fearful views about this group.

AWARENESS

Many students in nursing programs are unaware that there is a specialized body of knowledge in gerontological nursing. Throughout their programs they readily experience other areas of nursing, for example, medical/surgical nursing, maternal/child nursing, psychiatric/mental health nursing, and community health nursing. In most nursing curricula, however, content on the elderly is either embedded in courses with another major clinical focus or not incorporated at all. Ageist stereotypes and attitudes cannot be countered unless replaced with information and understanding. Students of nursing need to become cognizant of and informed about the wealth of information regarding older adults. This body of gerontological nursing knowledge can be included in nursing education in a number of ways.

In some institutions, gerontological nursing might be given division or department status. If this is not feasible in a particular academic structure, faculty members expert in gerontology within the academic setting should be identified and their expertise utilized, not only for student learning, but also for faculty development. Until most, if not all, nursing departments have such experts, external authorities need to be identified and utilized.

The "name it–teach it–evaluate it" principle should become a priority. It is essential that faculty members refer to gerontology/geriatrics throughout the curriculum and assimilate them into course materials. This necessitates that faculty themselves be knowledgeable about this content area. References such as Francis, Shenk, and Sokolovsky (1990), *Teaching about Aging: Interdisciplinary and Cross-Cultural Perspectives*, provides an excellent means for faculty to increase their own learning as well as offering a valuable resource for students. Additionally, increased testing of gerontologic knowledge must take place on both in-school and licensing exams.

Gerontology could become part of the research component of the curriculum, either as a segment of the research course or integrated throughout the curriculum. Every effort should be made to include research articles dealing with the elderly into mainstream teaching methodology. It is also helpful to have guest speakers who have conducted research with the elderly speak in research courses, professional issues courses, or clinical courses.

If learning resources are not current and readily available to students, the importance of gerontology is undermined and students will receive the impression that there is little to know about the elderly. The library must be well equipped with nursing and related gerontological textbooks and journals. Audiovisual and interactive teaching materials on the elderly should also be required learning aides.

Lastly, the media and public pressure must be employed to increase awareness and understanding of aging. Nursing faculty can be very instrumental in arranging public forums and enlisting those in the media to generate public relations campaigns to sensitize and enlighten the academic and broader community about the elderly. As Eyde and Rich (1983) state, "Old age should be publicly represented as one developmental phase within the human life span. Many of the secondary symptoms of pathological aging result from a variety of factors, including environmental deficiencies, stresses, and social stereotyping, that can be eliminated through remediation of the public mind" (pp. 211–212).

VOLUNTARY/ELECTIVE

When offered the opportunity to take elective courses on aging, many students retort, "I don't like it, I won't take your elective." Gerontological nursing content must be made mandatory in nursing curricula. Establishing and maintaining it as elective content dooms gerontological nursing content to failure, relegating it to lesser status than other areas of nursing. The message to students is that knowing about and practice with the elderly is nice but not necessary. Rather than seeing work with the elderly as an important and necessary aspect of nursing preparation, the field is perceived as tangential, irrelevant, and only for those who "like old people."

PROFESSIONAL/PRACTICE ISSUES

There are many perceptions about gerontological nursing that decrease its prestige and desirability as a practice specialty. In a survey of approximately 600 nurses (Glasspool & Arman, 1990), 41 percent of the respondents indicated that job satisfaction could be improved if there were greater acceptance of a gerontological specialty by others. The perpetuation of these notions in the profession often dissuades students from working with the elderly and from choosing the field as a career focus. This is most unfortunate as projections indicate that health-care providers will be spending approximately 70 percent of their patient-care time with those over 70 years of age (Brand & Gurenlian, 1989, cited in Mahoney, 1993). Yet of the 6243 graduates from master's programs in 1990, only 300, or 4.8 percent, specialized in gerontology (NLN, 1991).

Issues of prestige, salary, benefits, and job availability are considerations that influence students' career choices. Regrettably, gerontological nurses are often seen as having marginal status and prestige, being in unglamorous positions earning lower salaries, as compared with nurses in other specialties, gaining fewer benefits (e.g., tuition remission/reimbursement for graduate studies), and working exclusively in nursing homes. In addition, there is the persistent myth that gerontological nursing is "low-tech" and, hence, low status.

Again, there are a number of actions that can be taken to counteract these myths. Some of these have been discussed previously, such as increased exposure to all aspects of gerontology, attention to faculty attitudes in presenting gerontological material, and increased positive media exposure for gerontological nursing. Faculty also can stress the complexity and challenge of gerontic nursing care. Ebersole and Hess (1990) describe the role and function of gerontic nurses as "health advisors in the community, skillful technical care providers, scientific care planners, clinical nurse researchers, innovators and integrators" (p. 756). They go on to say that "This is not a field for nurses who wish to know 'more and more about less and less' or for those who are content to know 'less and less about more and more.' This is a field for holistic nurses, those who are willing to work with the whole client in an intensive relationship" (pp. 756–757). When one considers the implication of this role description, gerontic nursing appears to be one of the most complex and potentially creative/innovative practices that a nurse can undertake.

The variety of employment opportunities for gerontological nurses needs to be presented to students. Discussing and having students experience gerontic nursing practice in acute-care settings; long-term care, rehabilitation, and extended-care settings; day-care centers; residential settings; hospice facilities; homes; private practices; ambulatory clinics; retirement communities; social settings; and even organizations for the elderly, opens the eyes of students to the practice array and challenges available. Needless to say, having positive gerontological nurse role models speak about their practices enhances student enthusiasm for nursing with the older adult.

Regarding the perception that gerontological nursing is low-tech, it should be noted that the majority of hospital beds in acute-care facilities are occupied by elderly patients. Additionally, many of the conditions that were once treated in the hospital are now managed in the home, ergo, high-technology in-home care. Elderly patients in acute and critical care often have chronic illnesses that are uncontrolled and exacerbated by acute conditions. Yet many nurses are ill-prepared to care for the acutely ill elderly patient due to minimal knowledge of the needs of the aged or incorporation of age-appropriate interventions.

It is important for students to realize that "high-tech" also necessitates "high-cognitive" and "high-caring." Gioiella (1993) states, "Caring, concern with personal suffering, enhancing functional capacity, and use of palliative interventions will have much greater priority in elderly care in the future" (p. 105). An essential component of gerontological nursing is care of the whole person, and this demands tremendous professional nursing skills. As Ebersole and Hess insist, "Nurses have a particularly important role in the care of the critically ill aged. Nurses provide the integrating human contact so essential in sustaining the person caught in the web of machinery and complex treatments. . . . Manipulating the body systems is often a step toward cure, but the dissolution of illness is a process linked to the triad of care, coordination, and communication. . . . Equally important, critical-care nurses working with the aged must recognize that there is a difference between normal age changes and disease processes of aging, and that chronic illness complicates the care of the acutely ill" (pp. 765–766).

Finally, faculty should stress the inherent leadership role for nurses in elder care. Again quoting from Ebersole and Hess, "Coordination is critical in our highly specialized health-care delivery system. Nurses are in an ideal position to coordinate all aspects of care and assess the influence of microsystems and macrosystems on the patient and the patient's relationship to the system" (p. 766). Creativity, flexibility, a thorough knowledge base, familiarity with resources, imagination, and compassion are needed now—and will be increasingly so in the future—in caring for the vastly increasing numbers of elderly.

Another perception of gerontological nursing often held by students and nursing faculty is that there is too much regulation, with its concomitant development of burn-out. It is worthwhile for faculty to discuss with students the realities of clinical practice and effective strategies for dealing with regulatory aspects. Additionally, it must be emphasized that regulation and burnout are not restricted to geriatrics but are found increasingly in all practice foci.

"Caring for the elderly often requires a nurse to forego the reward of cure, [and] tolerate displaced anger of patients and families" (Ebersole & Hess, 1990, p. 761). Stress has become an inherent facet of much of nursing practice. The concept of "Care for the Caregiver" mentioned earlier bears repeating. The ability to care for others does not always translate to care for self. Caring for and about oneself and one's colleagues—and having that support reciprocated—is often the most effective means of avoiding burnout. The learning of assertive behaviors, stress-reduction strategies, and self care/peer support should be an integral component of all student nurses' education.

THE GERIATRIC MEDICAL MODEL

The exclusive use of the traditional medical model as a framework for assessment and care in geriatrics frequently adds to the stereotype of the elderly as frail, ill, and declining physically, mentally, and socially. Students of nursing must be helped to evaluate the limitations of this model for total care of the elderly. They must also be apprised of the distinct models for gerontological nursing practice. Unique opportunities for nurses in gerontic care including day care, home care, life care, and intergenerational programming and projects exist. Students need to be acquainted with the diverse roles of nurse practitioners and clinical nurse specialists in gerontological settings. And students should be informed of the emerging roles of gerontological nurses such as case management, home-care case management, geropsychiatric home care, telephone assessment and support, counseling and education, court investigation, architecture, and elder transportation.

The focus on interdisciplinary collaboration is becoming increasingly important in gerontological practice. This practice model allows students in various professions to collaborate in planning and delivery of care to the elderly. It also facilitates students' understanding about each others' roles, competencies, and responsibilities, fostering respect for one another and understanding of various disciplinary perspectives (Mariano, 1989, 1993). Interdisciplinary experiences strengthen nursing students' appreciation of the complexity of the elder population. Additionally, collaborative experiences demonstrate the integral role and contribution of nursing in assuring the well-being of the elderly.

Lastly, the role of gerontological nursing in both health-care reform and policy making requires accentuation for students. Gioiella (1993) notes that a central element of the emerging health-care system will be nursing centers, with the vast majority of clients in these centers being the well elderly. She indicates that the opportunity to model autonomous nursing capabilities for students in these centers is of prime import.

Palmore (1990) identified the jeopardy of positive stereotyping of the aged as better off socially, financially, and even physically then many in society. He contends that this form of ageism may proliferate public policies and procedures that disregard the unique needs of older persons. Matteson and McConnell (1988) aptly describe ageist policy when speaking of "compassionate ageism." This ageist attitude laid the foundation for many of the services and programs now in operation for the elderly without consideration of the differences among subgroups of elderly. " . . . [B]y obscuring the variation among the aged and simplifying the problems of a diverse group, it suggests that one solution applies to the entire group. Through statistical sleight of the hand, descriptions of the *plight* of the aged may later turn into descriptions of the *good fortune* of the aged when neither picture is entirely true. If such simplistic summaries are accepted by policy makers, it becomes acceptable to deny benefits to this group in times of economic hardship. . . . Once the problems of the aged have been reduced to a few simple problems, it is difficult to pull people out of the mindset that the aged are a homogeneous group with a relatively simple solution to their problems" (p. 485).

The above phenomenon creates a vicious cycle for the elderly. Estes and Binney (1991) claim that the elderly are often blamed for the health-care crisis and the broader economic crisis during times of economic hardship. They are also blamed for the poverty of children. This type of scapegoating of older persons distracts society from dealing with the very complicated and difficult issues at hand because it is easier for people (and policy makers) to contemplate and handle simplified problems.

Students of nursing must be made aware of the valuable role gerontological nurses can play in the policy arena. Gerontic nurses understand the individuality and heterogeneity of the elderly. As advocates for the elderly, gerontological nurses are essential in educating policy makers about the need to develop policy founded on criteria other than age and influencing policy which is sensitive to the unique needs of subgroups of older persons.

CONCLUSION

Ageism is prevalent in society. Its presence influences our attitudes toward, education about, practices with, and policies for the elderly. Overcoming ageism in nursing will only occur when faculty and the educational process provide the opportunity for nursing students to become aware of this prejudicial attitude and confront it directly. Student resistance to working with the elderly will be greatly diminished as students become cognizant of the challenges and valuable contributions of gerontological nursing.

REFERENCES

Barrett, E. (Ed.). (1990). *Visions of Rogers' science-based nursing.* New York: National League for Nursing.

Brand, M., & Gurenlian, J. (1989). Extending access to care: Preparing allied health practitioners for nontraditional settings. *Journal of Allied Health*, *18*(3), 261–270.

Burnside, I., & Schmidt, M. (1994). *Working with older adults: Group process and techniques* (3rd ed.). Boston: Jones & Bartlett Publishers.

Butler, R. (1969). Ageism: Another form of bigotry. *The Gerontologist*, *14*, 243–249.

Butler, R. (1975). *Why survive? Being old in America*. New York: McGraw-Hill.

Butler, R., Lewis, M., & Sunderland, T. (1991). *Aging and mental health positive psychosocial and biomedical approaches* (4th ed.). New York: Merrill Publishing.

Cook, B., & Pieper, H. (1985). The impact of nursing home clinical on attitudes toward working with the elderly. *Gerontology and Geriatrics Education*, *5*(4), 53–59.

Ebersole, P., & Hess, P. (1990). *Toward healthy aging: Human needs and nursing response* (3rd ed.). St. Louis: C. V. Mosby.

Estes, C., & Binney, E. (1991). The bio-medicalization of aging. In M. Minkler & C. Estes (Eds.), *Critical perspectives on aging: The political and moral economy of growing old*. Amityville, NY: Baywood Publishing Company.

Eyde, D., & Rich, J. (1983). *Psychological distress in aging*. Rockville, MD: Aspen.

Francis, D., Shenk, D., & Sokolovsky, J. (Eds.). (1990). *Teaching about aging: Interdisciplinary and cross-cultural perspectives*. St. Cloud State University, Minnesota: Association for Anthropology and Gerontology (AAGE).

Gioiella, E. (1993). Gerontological nursing education in the next millennium. *Gerontology and Geriatrics Education*, *13*(3), 99–106.

Glasspoole, L., & Arman, M. (1990). Knowledge, attitudes, and happiness of nurses working with gerontological patients. *Journal of Gerontological Nursing*, *16*(2), 11–13.

Kalish, R. (1979). The new ageism and the failure models: A polemic. *The Gerontologist*, *19*, 398–402.

Mahoney, D. (1993). Gerontology in the nursing curriculum: Evolution and issues. *Gerontology and Geriatrics Education*, *13*(3), 85–97.

Mariano, C. (1989). The case for interdisciplinary collaboration. *Nursing Outlook*, *37*(6), 285–288.

Mariano, C. (1993). *A model for nursing and medical school collaboration*. Paper presented at the Thirteenth Annual Stewart Conference on Research in Nursing, New York, NY.

Matteson, M. A., & McConnell, E. (1988). *Gerontological nursing concepts and practice*. Philadelphia: W. B. Saunders.

Matzo, M. (Guest Ed.). (1993). Integrating gerontology into the nursing curriculum. *Gerontology and Geriatrics Education, 13*(3), 3–106.

National League for Nursing. (1991). *Nursing datasource 1991: Leaders in the making—Graduate education in nursing* (vol. III). New York: NLN.

Nay-Brock, R. (1988). The impact of attitudes in care of the aged. *The Australian Nurses Journal, 17*(8), 15–17.

O'Reilly, M., & Kazanowski, M. (1993). Using change theory as a model to integrate gerontology into the nursing curriculum. *Gerontology and Geriatrics Education, 13*(3), 55–66.

Palmore, E. (1990). *Ageism: Negative and positive.* New York: Springer.

Rogers, M. (1986). Science of unitary human beings. In V. Malinski (Ed.), *Explorations on Martha Rogers' science of unitary human beings.* Norwalk, CT: Appleton-Century-Crofts.

Solomon, K. (1982). Social antecedents of learned helplessness in the health care setting. *The Gerontologist, 22*(3), 282–287.

Tiemann, K., & Stone, M. (1990). Teaching gerontology. In D. Francis, D. Shenk, & J. Sokolovsky (Eds.), *Teaching about aging: Interdisciplinary and cross-cultural perspectives.* St. Cloud University, Minnesota: Association for Anthropology and Gerontology (AAGE).

U.S. Senate Special Committee on Aging, The American Association of Retired Persons, The Federal Council on the Aging, and The U.S. Administration on Aging. (1991). *Aging America: Trends and projections.* Washington, DC: U.S. Department of Health and Human Services.

Chapter 6

INTEGRATED VERSUS COURSE-SPECIFIC PROGRAMS

Susan E. Sherman and Mary Burke

Historical discussions of curriculum development have included the important issue of integration versus course-specific approaches to content. Today, it still is true that any discussion of whether to integrate or not to integrate content in a curriculum raises supporters on both sides. Faculty who hold the view that content should not be integrated frequently use the rationale that they have the essential expertise and ability to teach the knowledge that students need. And, in many instances, at the time a faculty group realizes a new content area, like gerontology, needs to be in the curriculum, these experts are right. Right in the sense that, in fact, they may be the only content expert, and that their peers at that moment, are the novices. A second rationale for course-specific approaches is that responsibility for the course lies with one or two faculty. There are fewer time-consuming meetings, quicker negotiated resolutions, and fewer challenges as to the appropriateness of content and student-tracking methodologies.

Proponents on the side of integration of content, on the other hand, support the premise that curriculum should develop as a cohe-

---

This chapter reflects the efforts of the fifteen-member panel who participated in open and critical analysis of this issue.

sive whole, a unified state rather than a federation of course fiefdoms. These faculty are frequently challenged by working on a course planning team with faculty from areas of different specializations.

The inclusion of gerontological contents remains a challenge to dedicated faculty no matter how the curriculum is structured. One of the challenges faced by proponents of gerontological content are the faculty in the traditional acute-care areas (previously known as adult medical-surgical nursing) who defend their time and content choices with arguments that are reality oriented. Arguments such as, they are already caring for more elderly individuals in their clinical courses; they have already accommodated their course content to the shifting demographics; they have far too little time as it is to add additional content or to give up critical content, are always presented. Traditional arguments for course-specific approaches also include the assurance that all students will be provided with similar learning experiences and an opportunity to engage in this learning with an expert practitioner faculty member, and one who is passionate about the content. For faculty members who frequently are evaluated based on course-specific models, individual accountability is much easier maintained in nonintegrated courses.

For proponents of gerontological content integration, these arguments are the most difficult to refute. Yet, not to engage in just this discussion maintains the status quo. Gerontological nursing experts have the task of convincing peers that just because they are "dealing" with elders in clinical settings, it does not necessarily follow that the care is appropriate and specific to this population; and just because people are being cared for at a point in time, it does not necessarily follow that the caregiver sees the elder person in the greater context of their life. The challenge to gerontological nursing experts is to convince both students and peers that care outcomes, though not dramatic in many instances, provide the caregiver with opportunities to observe subtle changes, and, that, these subtleties should be as valued by nurses as the dramatic ones that occur in ICUs.

These different positions frequently lead to discussions of two important questions for all faculty to address. What should be integrated? What knowledge skills and values do we believe all students should have the opportunity to master? The anticipated faculty involvement in answering these questions may cause some schools to shrink from the task. Additionally, accreditation outcomes criteria may introduce hesitancy in faculties, which will inhibit their ability to change appropriately.

If a faculty accepts the challenge of providing the knowledge, skills, and attitudes necessary to provide safe and effective care to the elderly client, their work should begin by carrying out a content analyses of content taught in the curriculum to verify the importance of each content area and to find duplication of content and gaps. They will need to accept and invest in the underlying philosophy of the lifespan approach as a critical determinant in curriculum development. Agreement on what concepts are to be integrated will have to be reached, and how these concepts will be approached across clinical rotations will have to occur.

This is a time-consuming process and faculty who engage in this activity will need the support of program administrators. Inservices should be developed to allow discussions and understandings to emerge about ageism and the general societal view of aging; understandings about the pre-existing conception and personal views of aging that both faculty and students bring to the elderly person's bedside; discussions about the expanding definitions of health, healthy elderly and function; and finally, discussions about semantics, the words we choose to define clients, elders, and ourselves. Faculty also will need support in living with the ambiguity of these discussions as new ideas take time to emerge, grab hold and conceptualizations occur. Without such support little change will come. The outcomes of understandings (new comfort zones) will not happen rapidly, but rather through the dedicated hard work of committed faculty.

It is incumbent upon nursing leaders who understand the process of faculty development. Support of a shift in focus for both State Boards of Nursing and national accreditation standards that value this faculty process as both necessary and critical for ongoing curriculum development needs to occur. As this process of shifting values begins, it is expected that a dysequilibrium between philosophy, course outlines, and clinical outcomes will occur.

Given the discussion on pedagogical approaches, the important area for student mastery remains understanding of the elderly client. This vision of the elder as a unique individual, a person who brings to the care setting a lifetime of experiences and strengths that are both physiological and psychosocial, should be encouraged. This understanding can be best garnered by interaction with a well elder and the environment where they reside.

The responsibility for all faculty in making the critical decision between integrated versus course-specific content lies in the gaining of an adequate knowledge base to make an appropriate decision for the time and the program of learning. Less importance should be placed on how content is approached or where it is placed. Rather, how it is valued by all faculty and in turn by the students as a critical component of the nursing curriculum, is key to its inclusion now and in the future.

Chapter 7

LESSONS FROM SUCCESSFUL CURRICULUM MODELS

Susan Sherman

A review of successful curricula models designed for integration of gerontological content into nursing programs—course- or program-specific—has inherent difficulty in that the measures of curriculum paradigms and the measures of success have not been clearly defined and subjected to consensus. A review of the literature of gerontological content in nursing curricula might lead to the conclusion that most of the work has been conducted, through federal and private funding, and as such the successful outcomes seem to be related to the length of the grant period. The conclusion that can be made about successful projects is that, in most instances, they can only be measured locally, in one school, with one faculty. To date, there is no metaanalysis or overriding set of voluntary accreditation standards that specifically require curricula to address gerontological content. Consequently, there is no mandate for curricular change. Without such mandates, the struggle for possession of the curriculum between and among individual faculty continues.

Much was done throughout the 1980s to lay the foundation for consensus and change. Multiple attempts to define essential curriculum content occurred, as evidenced in the work of Brower (1985, 1988), Gunter and Estes (1979), Gioella (1986), Schwartz (1978), Waters (1991), Tagliareni (1991), Burke and Sherman (1993). Nursing organizations, too, supported the need to increase content and clinical practice with the elderly. The AACN, ANA, and NLN published statements and passed resolutions to this end. The Robert Wood Johnson and the W.K. Kellogg foundations have actively supported university and community-college projects that examined work roles, competencies, and curricular shifts, as has the Division of Nursing, Bureau of Health Professions. Over a ten-year period, Ross Laboratories sponsored multiple nursing conferences under the umbrella of the NLN, and published their outcomes (NLN, 1988). With the support of the Merck Company Foundation, this book contributes to the effort to examine and agree on gerontological content for nursing education. Given the demographics of our nation, this effort could not be more timely.

The majority of acute-care, long-term care, and home-care clients are elderly. Comprehensive services required by this population include a focus on maintenance, rehabilitation, and support in decline. The skills required by nurses caring for the elderly include a strong knowledge base in science and theory, coupled with compassion and patience. Nurses will require a new way of thinking about the elderly to manage the services required by this population. Pockets of gerontological content inserted into individual nursing courses and taught by the single expert on the faculty will not meet this need. Curricula developed autonomously within individual colleges and universities will not meet this need. Commitment to similarity in curricular goals is needed, as is dialogue between and among faculty and practitioners. The disparity of content emphasis in programs today may be attributed to a lack of prepared faculty as much as a lack of interest. Johnson and Connelly (1990) aptly refer to the "self-taught" faculty as the reason that a comprehensive and deep understanding of gerontology is not common. Yet they state this cannot be the sole reason that inclusion of gerontology content does not occur. Nursing faculty need to become specialized generalists in gerontology. Projects such as the Teaching Nursing Home and Community College–Nursing Home Partnership can provide guidance to us. Lessons learned by faculty should be widely disseminated in attempts to understand the processes and products of faculty change. Content outlined in the NLN publication *Gerontology in the Nursing*

Curriculum (1992) should be reviewed. Opportunities such as attending geriatric education center programs should be maximized.

Lessons learned in the past should be the foundation upon which we build the future. Let us examine some of these lessons.

LESSONS FROM THE ROBERT WOOD JOHNSON (RWJ) TEACHING NURSING HOME PROJECT

In 1987, this project brought together 11 universities and 12 nursing homes to produce models for joint efforts between education and practice. Jointly funded by the RWJ Foundation and the American Academy of Nursing, it sought to pool personnel as well as physical and financial resources to the mutual benefit of the institutions and society. The program provided an opportunity for schools of nursing to establish clinical affiliations with nursing homes, with some faculty in positions involving direct responsibility for patient care, serving as nurse practitioners, clinical specialists, assistant directors of nursing, and directors of quality assurance. In some instances, faculty contracted for research or more traditional roles as clinical instructors for students.

The models developed through this project resulted in numerous successes. Still, difficulties with the lack of resources in these settings, personnel, the highly regulated nature of the environment, and the lack of rewards in a university environment for curriculum work, not to mention the small number of faculty committed to gerontology, made the curriculum impact less than revolutionary. Mezey, Lynaugh, and Cartier (1989) reports that mechanisms to maintain faculty enthusiasm remained elusive given the turnover of nursing home staff coupled with the other variables such as environment, lower pay, and lower status. Nevertheless, a valuable outcome of the project was the realization that the nursing-home environment is an ideal setting for students to determine the efficacy of their therapeutic strategies, in a nurse-managed, consultative, and collaborative environment.

The resulting curriculum models, sustained in some schools and not in others, were diverse, with more emphasis on advanced practice and less on generic education. The content integration would most likely be characterized as course-specific and not consistent with the curriculum of the 1980s, which valued technology and more visible nursing roles.

LESSONS LEARNED IN THE W. K. KELLOGG– NURSING HOME PARTNERSHIP PROJECT

Funded initially in 1986 and again in 1990, this project promised to show how the (then) 778 associate-degree nursing programs dispersed throughout urban and rural America could influence nursing-home care and influence the redirection of curriculum nationally. Six schools served as demonstration sites. Taking some initial lessons from the federation of schools in the RWJ project, one of the initial activities of the NHP project was to engage in a DACUM (Developing a Curriculum) process with nurses who worked in nursing homes to find out exactly what their job responsibilities were on a day-to-day basis. The DACUM (Burke & Sherman, 1993) resulted in over 300 specific statements, which when analyzed evolved into the four competency categories called "Best Taught in the Nursing Home." These categories were: perform assessment of the resident, practice rehabilitation nursing skills, manage the living environment, and exhibit management skills. Within these four categories, 25 specific competencies provide curriculum guidance. As this project evolved and faculty in the six project schools developed knowledge and comfort with caring for the frail elderly, it became apparent that a positive experience with the elderly at the beginning of a nursing curriculum was essential for students. Led by models developed at Valencia Community College in a well-elder experience, the ADN program prototype is a first-semester, well-elder experience, followed by integration of content throughout the curriculum, with a capstone four- to five-week experience in the nursing home in the final semester of the program. It is of interest that the evolution of this curriculum has resulted in prototypes of clients, all of whom are over 65, being classroom models for teaching nursing using case studies. A recent national survey of all ADN schools demonstrates that over 300 programs nationally have adopted many of the concepts from the partnership project (Newslink, Winter, 1994). One reason given for the success of this project is the permission for faculty to learn, to experiment, and to share both successes and failures. As with the Teaching Nursing Home Project, faculty resistance to change was, and continues to be, the most difficult barrier to overcome.

LESSONS FROM THE GERIATRIC EDUCATION CENTERS

These centers, federally funded in the 1980s, provided valuable learning to interested faculty in both content and interdisciplinary studies. They were, and are, an important resource for all healthcare professionals, offering credit and noncredit courses. Their success, though, is individual, in that a motivated faculty member, usually only one or two, would attend, leading to course-specific changes.

LESSONS FROM THE GERONTOLOGIC NURSING EDUCATION CONTINUING CARE PROJECT, GEORGETOWN UNIVERSITY

In 1990, 18 leaders in gerontologic nursing practice, administration, and education met for an intensive two-day, group-facilitated consensus project to develop competency statements for BSN and master's graduates. Published by the NLN, in *Gerontology in the Nursing Curriculum* (1993), these statements speak both to professional practice roles and nursing process expectations. They have the potential to serve as either course or curriculum guidelines, but as yet no follow-up on their use has been reported in the literature.

It should be noted that nurses have followed and participated in other important studies, including the early work of Midwest Alliance in Nursing (MAIN) and the more recent Southern Regional Education Board (SREB), Teaching Gerontological Nursing in Southern States. A recent article by Brower and Yurchuck (1993) examines the dilemma of "to integrate or separate" gerontological content. On the side of integration falls:

1. Emphasis on the continuum of care
2. Repeated exposure to the problems of older adults
3. Improved student attitudes about elderly people

The separation argument includes:

1. Elimination of the segregation of older adults
2. Insurance of the important content
3. Clinical emphasis taught by experts

Those who argue against integration fear that content is lost and-never-found-again if all faculty are not committed to ensuring its presence. This potential is real, given that faculty who are not specialists in gerontology are, and should be expected to be, novices in this area. Textbooks frequently do not help students or faculty, and arguments are still put forth that specific content is not reflected in NCLEX-RN exams and accreditation standards. Perhaps these reasons have some credibility. Johnson and Connelly (1990), in a listing of factors influencing lack of gerontological nursing content suggest seven areas:

1. Lack of demand for inclusion
2. Lack of gerontological nursing faculty
3. Lack of clinical role models
4. Multiplicity of topics
5. Rapidly changing knowledge base
6. Approval and accreditation processes
7. Licensure (NCLEX-RN)

I would like to conclude my remarks with a personal comment about these seven categories. Our own experience in the W.K. Kellogg Community College-Nursing Home Partnership project supports the validity of many of these concerns. It is critical that we recognize that all faculty need some expertise in gerontology. In the meantime, we cannot wait for exemplary role models to emerge. As faculty we are the role models for our students—if not as experts, then as partners in learning with them. We have the obligation to design curricula that respond to the demographics of our society.

REFERENCES

Brower, H. T. (1985). Knowledge competencies in gerontological nursing. In *Overcoming the bias of ageism in long-term care* (pp. 55–82). New York: National League for Nursing.

Brower, H. T. (1988). Knowledge competencies in gerontological nursing. In *Strategies for Long-Term Care* (pp. 135–161). New York: National League for Nursing (Pub. # 20-2231).

Brower, H. T., & Yurchuck, E. R. (April, 1993). Teaching gerontological nursing in Southern states. *Nursing and Health Care, 14*, 4.

Burke, M., & Sherman, S. (Eds.). (1993). *Gerontological nursing: Issues and opportunities for the twenty-first century.* New York: National League for Nursing Press (pub. # 14-2510).

Community College Nursing Home Partnership. (1994, Winter). *Newslink,* Community College at Philadelphia, p. 3.

Gerontology in the Nursing Curriculum. (1992). New York: National League for Nursing Press. (Pub. # 14-2506).

Gioiella, E. C. (Ed.). (1986). *Gerontology in the professional curriculum.* New York: National League for Nursing. (pub. # 15-2151).

Gunter, L. M., & Estes, C. (1979). *Education for geriatric nursing.* New York: Springer.

Johnson, M. A., & Connelly, J. R. (1990). *Nursing and gerontology: Status report.* Washington, DC: Association for Gerontology in Higher Education

Mengel, A., Simson, S., Sherman, S., & Waters, V. (1991). Essential Factors in a Community College–Nursing Partnership. *Journal of Gerontologic Nursing, 16*, 11, 26–31.

Mezey, N. D., Lynaugh, J. E., & Cartier, N. M. (Eds.). (1989). *Nursing home and nursing care: Lessons from the teaching nursing home.* New York: Springer.

Moses, D. V. (1968). Geriatrics in the baccalaureate nursing curriculum. *Nursing Outlook, 16*, 41–44.

National League for Nursing. (1988). *Strategies for long-term care.* New York. National League for Nursing. (pub.# 20–2231).

Schwartz, D. (1978). Public health nursing's responsibilities for care of the aged. *Bulletin of the New York Academy of Medicine, 54,* 555.

Tagliareni, E., Sherman, S., Waters, V., & Mengel, V. (1991). Participatory Clinical Education: Reconceptualizing the clinical learning environment. *Nursing and Health Care, 12*(5), 248–263.

Waters, V. (1991). *Teaching Gerontology.* New York: National League for Nursing (pub. # 15-2411).

Part II

Approaches to Specific Content Areas

Chapter 8

PHYSIOLOGICAL CHANGES IN AGING

Mary Burke and Susan Sherman

The ability to differentiate between normal age-related changes and pathology is dependent on a knowledge base of the physiological changes that are inherent in the process of aging. Therefore, physiological age-related changes are important aspects of every nursing curriculum.

The human condition dictates that chronological aging is a universal experience and physiological changes always accompany chronological aging. How a person responds to the aging process is a result of a myriad of factors, such as personality, culture, genetic endowment, and health state. This chapter discusses the universality of aging as well as the diversity of the aging experience.

The challenge to gerontological nursing educators is to impart the knowledge base of what are the human physiological age changes that are universally experienced. It is essential that faculty and students acknowledge that there are irreversible, nondesirable, age-related physiological changes (e.g., bone loss). Students must recognize that these changes do not incapacitate healthy older people. Nursing faculty should stress the utmost respect for the courage and versatility of older adults as they respond to and compensate for physiological changes. It is by allowing students to view aging in this manner that will facilitate their appreciation for the dignity and diversity of each elder person. The ability to examine what is meant by the mature, healthy adult in a physiological sense will assist the student to begin to appreciate and recognize normal age-related changes.

BIOLOGICAL PRINCIPLES OF AGING

To assist students in understanding physiological aging it is helpful to teach a principled biological approach. This approach facilitates an understanding of biological aging but preserves the importance of physiological diversity among older people.

Biological principles of healthy aging:

(A) Differences between people. Principle: all organisms do not age at the same rate.
(B) Differences within the person. Principle: all organ systems in one organism do not age at the same rate.

Examples of differences in aging:

(A) All 70-year-old people do not experience the aging process in the same way.
(B) Within each 70-year-old person, organs (such as the heart, brain) do not age at the same rate.

A teaching strategy to illustrate example A is to show a slide of a number of 6-to-8-month-old infants. Have the student discuss the physiologic similarities of this age group: the number of similarities in function as a result of physiological development, such as, the inability to walk (neurological and musculoskeletal development), or talk (higher cortical development), will highlight the lack of diversity in physiological development at this young age.

Principle B is illustrated using a slide showing a group of 80-year-old people. The diversity in appearance and function should allow the student to discuss how the lived experience of multiple years affects function and physiological development. A second slide can show older senior Olympians or runners in juxtaposition to a sedentary older person sitting on a park bench. This leads students to realize the effects over time of an active, healthy lifestyle.

BIOLOGICAL THEORY

After development of a biological principle approach, faculty can introduce biological theories of aging. A genetic and nongenetic discussion of the theories assists the students in their understanding of the theories and their ability to integrate this knowledge into their clinical experiences.

The importance of family history will highlight some aspects of genetic influences on physiological development and on the susceptibility to certain conditions. Nongenetic theories will heighten the student's understanding of environmental aspects and the results of a healthy versus an abusive lifestyle.

In introducing the student to biological aging theory faculty need to acknowledge the diversity of opinion and the lack of universal support for any one theory. The premise of the compression of morbidity proposed by Fries (1988) should be introduced at this point in the student's exposure to gerontological nursing. The premise is that the lifespan is finite and the morbidity from chronic disease can be postponed by healthy lifestyles and by the reallocation of resources in research and technology from life extension to postponement of chronic disease. As a consequence, the survivorship curve of aging will change from a declining line to a rectangularity of the aging experience. This change will allow the coming generations of older adults to enjoy more years of vitality and good health than in the past.

In support of genetic theories, studies have shown that in vitro cell proliferation has a finite number of cell divisions. Each cell has about 50 cell divisions within the cell's lifetime. These studies also demonstrate that young cell tissue has a greater number of cell divisions than those of older cell tissue (Hayflick, 1985).

The Cross-Linking theory assists students to understand the loss of tissue elasticity that influences many of the physical changes experienced by the aging adult. This theory suggests that a chemical reaction influences cellular division. Changes occur in collagen and new fibers are produced and cross-link chemically causing increased density. The results of these changes cause elastin to become less efficient and more rigid, leading to a reduction in pulmonary compliance. This theory also explains many of the age-related changes seen in the older population such as a change in skin turgor which results from the loss of elastin's flexibility.

The increase in susceptibility to infections and certain diseases such as cancer can be partially explained through an understanding of the decline in the immune system. The body's ability to effectively produce T-cells declines, bone marrow stem cells lose efficiency, and the weight of the thymus declines. These changes lend support to a biological approach to aging.

The nongenetic theories are developed around the role of the environment as a causative factor in the process of aging. The effects of radiation, the ingestion of substances that are harmful such as lead, mercury, and the breathing of fumes of pollution such as tobacco are examples of environmental effects that influence the aging process. It should become obvious to students that there is no one biological theory that can explain all the complexities of aging but that elements of each theory have merit and can aid nurses in their understanding of biological aging.

Functional Results of Normal Physiological Change

Function is the hallmark of a healthy old age. The ability to adapt to physiological changes is one of the challenges of aging. The importance of limited physical reserve and slowed neurological response time to the demands of daily life need to be emphasized to students.

One teaching strategy is an assignment that has the student observe elderly people walking across a busy traffic intersection. The need for speed in crossing the street safely and the rise of pedestrian injuries in the elderly population will highlight the relationship among function, physiological change, and susceptibility. The need for physical reserve in daily life can be demonstrated in many ways. Suggestions include showing elderly persons running to catch a bus, shoveling snow, carrying groceries. The possibilities are great. Faculty need only to look in their geographical areas and let students discuss all the challenges elderly people meet on a daily basis that are a result of physiological changes.

The ability to understand the importance of function in daily life needs to be emphasized in any gerontological experience.

Assessment

Functional assessment of community-dwelling elderly provides an excellent opportunity to assist students to appreciate the challenges physiological changes demand of the older adult. The use of validated scales is encouraged to allow the student to value the scientific development that is a hallmark of geriatric assessment.

Observation of elderly clients is an excellent teaching opportunity to assist students in analyzing the effects of normal age-related changes. Changes in skin, nails, hair color, posture, and gait are all observable characteristics that have a physiological base that are related to normal changes inherent in the aging process.

Physical assessment core courses need to include normal age changes. The assessment of mental status of the elderly person is a complex task. Students need to be aware that asking simple questions of orientation does not suffice as an accurate assessment of mental status. In-depth assessment of mental status using validated assessment tools needs to be a significant part of a course in assessment of older adults. Normal physiological changes will affect an older adult's response time, and particularly if the environment is stressful. Recall of events may be slowed and the elderly person may be labeled as forgetful. These slowed responses are within a range of normal for an elderly person and should not cause any inappropriate labeling of the person.

The importance of ethnic consideration, literacy abilities, and level of hearing acuity are also factors that influence responses to mental status examinations. It is important to be sure the older person is comfortable and not intimidated by the questions. But the students must realize that it is not appropriate to cue the person for the answers to questions. Changes in mental status may be transient and signs of stress, but they may also be early harbingers of decline in mental status caused by an unrecognized disease process. Students should learn to perform as accurate an assessment of mental status changes as they learn about physical assessment techniques.

DIFFERENTIATION BETWEEN NORMAL AGING CHANGES AND CHRONIC ILLNESS

In the past many physiological changes that result from chronic illness were attributed to normal aging. Recent studies have demonstrated that aspects of cardiac and kidney function thought to result from aging were actual disease processes. On the other hand, aging does increase a person's susceptibility to disease and to death. The issue for gerontological nursing educators is to successfully prepare the graduate to be able to provide holistic nursing care to the elder population.

Knowledge of the older adult's response to the disease process is essential to be able to provide appropriate care. Most students have learned that a myocardial infarction is always manifested in the patient by severe chest pain. Gerontological nursing educators not only have to teach content relative to the older adult, but they have to help students unlearn information that had been presented as also indisputable scientific fact accompanied by unquestioning faith. An older adult may indeed have cardiac ischemia with none of the typical clinical manifestations. It is essential that modern-day nurses be educated to ask questions and to seek answers to their questions through scientific inquiry.

Because of physiological change interacting with the disease process, elderly persons' responses are blunted so that atypical responses are common in older people. Infection may be present in the absence of fever and the only symptom may be a change in the person's mental status. Severe chest pain may be completely nonexistent in an older person who is experiencing a severe myocardial infarction. Again, a general malaise with changes in mental status may be the only symptom that is expressed by the older person. Thyroid disease, urinary tract infections, and adverse drug reactions will have atypical presentations.

The physiological aspects of the aging process are highly influenced by genetic, lifestyle, and environmental factors. In spite of the high degree of variations in individual response to age-related physiological changes, students need to be knowledgeable of the normal changes plus the effect the changes may have on the older person's ability to carry on the activities of daily life.

REFERENCES

Fries, J. F. (1988). Aging, illness, and health policy: Implications of the compression of morbidity. *Perspective Biological Medicine, 31,* 407–423.

Hayflick, L. (1985). Theories of biological aging. *Experimental Gerontology, 20,* 145.

Chapter 9

PSYCHIATRIC MENTAL HEALTH CONTENT FOR GERONTOLOGICAL NURSING EDUCATION

Carol M. Musil and May L. Wykle

The essential goals of teaching geriatric mental health content to nursing students are to impart knowledge, shape attitudes, and foster skills that will promote the health of older adults, regardless of whether the content is integrated throughout the curriculum, is specific to geriatric or psychiatric nursing curricula, or both. Certainly, psychiatric principles should be integrated into the gerontology content. Ideally, intra- and interdisciplinary integration of gerontology content into the total program is suggested, although some faculty have found that students may have difficulty identifying specific geropsychiatric knowledge when taught in this manner. Further, the faculty may not have the necessary gerontology background or find time to add the material in their specialty courses. It has been demonstrated that content knowledge and clinical skills of geriatric mental health warrant their own time. The commitment of all faculty is essential to the success of an integrated program.

This chapter will review essential content areas for geriatric mental health education. Four content areas need to be considered: (1) mental health; cognitive disorders, including delirium and dementias; (2) psychiatric disorders, including anxiety, depression, paranoia, and chronic mental illness; (3) substance abuse disorders;

and (4) cognitive disorders. Clinical placement for a gerospychiatric student experience will also be discussed.

MENTAL HEALTH

The majority of older persons experience relatively good mental health rather than mental illness. In fact, older adults have lower rates of affective, anxiety, and substance use disorders than younger persons (Regier et al., 1984). Clearly, the mental health of older adults underscores their successful aging, and frequently mental health stays the same or may even improve (Haug, Belgrave, & Gratton, 1984). Mental health issues of elders must be taught, preferably as a continuum concept, in addition to the traditional focus on psychopathology. The promotion and maintenance of mental health needs to be woven through all of gerontologic education. The psychiatric/ mental health integrator model in which psychosocial concepts are taught throughout the program, but actual mental illness is taught in various ways at appropriate times, is useful. In many programs, one expert faculty is used throughout the curriculum. An alternate model is one in which core psychosocial concepts are taught to all students in the junior year, and concurrently, students receive specialty knowledge in a clinical course, such as psychiatric nursing.

Either integration during the educational program or a core content track can be successful. Expense, faculty expertise, and teaching load are considered when making these decisions. Incorporating a variety of teaching strategies will provide opportunities for students to explore a range of geropsychiatric/mental health issues, such as adaptive systems, crisis intervention, and developmental stages. Teaching/learning methods might include journals, case studies, role playing, games, and student-generated videos, all of which provide ample opportunities for analysis of mental health problems of older adults.

PSYCHIATRIC DISORDERS

Although many older adults enjoy relatively good mental health, problems of anxiety or depression may interfere with life satisfaction and maximum functioning. Individuals who have chronic mental illness are also likely to be underserved. The issues with acute or chronic mental illness are further complicated by the fact that older adults are less likely than younger persons to seek help for mental health problems from mental health providers, although primary care practitioners provide an estimated one-half to three-fourths of the mental health care to this population (Burns & Taube, 1990). While these providers have generally been physicians, nurses in both inpatient and outpatient settings can make important contributions to the identification and treatment patterns of older adults experiencing mental illness. The need for adequate preparation in the area of geropsychiatric illness suggests directions for educational programs in nursing, especially in the development of geropsychiatric nurse practitioners.

Depression

Although it is commonly thought that psychiatric disorders, particularly depression, are more prevalent among older than younger persons, the Epidemiologic Catchment Area Project (ECA) data suggest otherwise (Myers et al., 1984). Based on data from 4 ECA sites, the prevalence of major depression in adults over the age of 65 was reported to be less than 0.95%, whereas the prevalence for those 64 and younger was 1½ to 3 times higher (George, Blazer, Winfield-Laird, Leaf, & Fischbach, 1988). In a closer look at depressive symptoms in the elderly, Blazer, Hughes, and George (1987) found that approximately 27% of 1300 adults over age 60 in the ECA study reported a variety of depressive symptoms. While only 0.8% of the total sample was eligible for a diagnosis of major depressive disorder based on *Diagnostic and Statistical Manual of Mental Disorders* (DSM-III) criteria, 19% experienced mild dysphoria, 4% mild depression, 2% dysthymia, and 1.2% mixed anxiety and depression. In a review of other epidemiologic surveys of mental illness, Anthony and Aboraya (1992) concur that estimates for major depression in the 65-plus population generally fall within the 0.5% to 2.0% range. The lower rates of diagnosed depressive disorders may reflect the presence of widespread but relatively mild depressive symptoms among older adults. More problematic is the likelihood that some criteria and instruments to measure depression in older adults are not "age fair" and hence underreport the extent of depression among certain segments of elders. Often depression in older adults is dismissed as normal aging when the individual's quality of life could be improved with treatment.

The prevalence of depressive symptoms in the elderly commands attention from those planning nursing curricula. Older adults certainly experience more losses of significant others, health, activities, and other outlets than do most younger adults. They may be more prone to experience grief reactions, although some authors, such as Neugarten (1969) suggest that such reactions may be less likely if the events occur "on time" as an expected life event.

Those with depressive symptoms are more likely to be women, unmarried or widowed, of lower socioeconomic status, and to have physical health problems, more stressful life events, and a less supportive social network (Blazer, Hughes, & George, 1987; Krause, 1991; NIH Consensus Development Conference Statement, 1991; Wykle & Musil, 1993). Suicide remains one of the top 10 causes of death for those over 65. Older persons commit 17% of all suicides, and tend to choose lethal means to do so (Koenig & Blazer, 1992). Elderly persons with mental illness or poor physical health and men are at greater risk for suicide attempts.

Importantly, depression and physical illness often co-occur. Depression may be a concomitant feature of medical or neurologic disorders such as stroke, hypothyroidism, Parkinson's disease, and delirium or dementia. In other cases, symptoms of decreased cognitive function, such as apathy, inattention, and impaired memory or abstract ability, may be indicative of pseudodementia or dementia syndrome of depression (Berezin, Liptzin, & Salzman, 1988). Although depressed persons of all ages are likely to show problems with memory and concentration, these impairments may be apparent when testing only the most severely depressed (LaRue, Yang, & Osato, 1992). Thus, distinctions between depression secondary to illness, a masked depression that presents with physical symptoms, and physiological, metabolic, or pharmacologically induced depression must be made since these have important treatment and prognostic implications (Koenig & Blazer, 1992).

Anxiety Disorders

The lifetime prevalence for anxiety disorders approaches 15% (Regier et al., 1988) although adults 65 and over have markedly lower rates of anxiety disorders, 3.6% compared with approximately 5% for all other age groups. Similar ratios exist for panic disorders (0.1% compared with 0.3–0.5%), phobic disorders (3% compared with 3.5%–5%), and obsessive–compulsive disorders, which are half as prevalent in those over 45 as in younger adults. Sheikh (1992) suggests that a much higher number of older adults experience clinically significant anxiety symptoms, 10%–20%, with 2%–10% of older men and women likely to experience phobias. Not uncommonly, anxiety disorders begin after a serious life event which is interpreted as a threat to one's future well-being. For instance, a fall resulting in hip fracture may contribute to a subsequent fear of falling that reaches phobic proportions.

Another anxiety disorder, obsessive–compulsive disorder, is marked by obsessive thoughts about body functioning or morbid fears, and compulsive rituals to deal with the associated anxiety. In other cases, anxiety about cognitive changes and efforts to compensate for these may stimulate obsessive–compulsive rituals. There is some evidence to suggest that obsessive–compulsive behavior and decreased cognitive function both may be associated with a decrease in serotonin and norepinephrine (Anthony & Aboraya, 1992), although additional research to examine this connection is underway.

An important consideration with anxiety disorders is their association with physical symptoms. For instance, some physical conditions such as hypothyroidism, myocardial infarction, and hypoxia may cause anxiety-like symptoms (Gurian & Goisman, 1993; Jenike, 1989; Sheikh, 1992). Further, there remains some suggestion that anxiety contributes to certain medical conditions such as asthma or ulcers. On the psychological front, anxiety syndromes in elderly persons may be difficult to distinguish since anxiety is thought to coexist in many cases of depression, and conversely a depressed mood may be secondary to anxiety. Although the overall prevalence may be lower, anxiety disorders can be even more difficult to deal with for older persons who may have fewer supports and coping options than younger persons.

Paranoia

About 4% of older persons may develop paranoia and suspiciousness. In some cases, such mistrust and suspiciousness might have a basis in reality, but the fears have become exaggerated (McDougall, 1994). Frequently a sensory loss, such as a hearing impairment, may contribute to lack of trust and suspiciousness, or realistic fears about being the victim of crime might become magnified and reach delusional proportions. Not uncommonly, paranoia develops toward significant others around issues of belonging, possession, and control, particularly when the individual is isolated. Occasionally, paranoia that others are out to harm one results in refusal to take medication or participate in medical treatment. As Rabins (1992) points out, however, such complaints may be valid, as in cases of elder abuse, but finding corroborating or refuting evidence will be a necessary, although sensitive issue. Delusions, suspiciousness, and paranoia all may be associated with brain disorders such as Alzheimer's disease. In fact, some researchers (Erkinjuntti, Wikstrom, Palo, & Autio, 1986) suggest that the development of a delirium from an acute illness or reaction to a medication may signal the presence of underlying dementia. Teaching nursing students about the many aspects of dealing with paranoid patients is critical, especially for those who will be working in the community.

Schizophrenia

Schizophrenia typically emerges in the late teens or the early 20s, although some cases of late-onset schizophrenia may occur, most commonly in women. Older chronic schizophrenics are likely to exhibit fewer symptoms than younger counterparts and to have made accommodations for living with their illness; many may be counted among the ranks of the homeless. Some who carry the label "schizophrenic" may have been misdiagnosed when younger, and thus accurate history-taking is essential. According to DSM-III criteria, schizophrenia must be diagnosed before age 40, although Rabins (1992) indicates that late-onset schizophrenia does appear, primarily in individuals who were isolated, not married, and childless, suggesting a history of unusual predisposing personality characteristics. The symptoms of late-onset schizophrenia are similar to early-onset schizophrenia, although patients' affect may be less flat and hallucinations may be more florid, including not just auditory but visual, olfactory, tactile, and gustatory hallucinations as well (Rabins, 1992). Since nonauditory hallucinations may be associated with other conditions, including toxic psychoses, careful medical and psychological examination is necessary.

SUBSTANCE ABUSE DISORDERS

Until the early 1990s, little attention was focused on substance use and abuse by older adults. There are few reliable data about this problem which had gone virtually unstudied until recently. The ECA data suggest that 3%–4% of men over age 65 have an alcohol problem, and that drug abuse and dependence are infrequent. When considering the prevalence of substance use, differences in behavior patterns between cohort groups are particularly important, perhaps even more than in other psychiatric illnesses. For example, current cohorts of older adults are more likely to use alcohol, tobacco, benzodiazapenes, and sleeping pills rather than illegal drugs. Cohorts of elders who turned 21 during prohibition have lower prevalence rates of alcohol use than do younger cohorts of elderly adults (Atkinson, Ganzini, & Bernstein, 1992). Since prevalence data on substance use in all age groups is unreliable, there are few data to suggest how cohort effects and age effects influence prevalence rates of substance use by elderly adults.

With age, there is greater biological sensitivity to alcohol and a heightened neuropharmacodynamic effect (Atkinson et al., 1992; Vogel-Sprott & Barrett, 1984). Nurses need to develop clinical interviewing and assessment skills to evaluate moderate alcohol use patterns in addition to screening for alcoholism. Moderate alcohol use in elders may have implications for their health and coping during acute and chronic hospitalizations and for their functioning in the community.

COGNITIVE DISORDERS

It is estimated that between 4%–8% of those over 65 and 20%–35% of those in their 80s experience some degree of dementia (Evans et al., 1989; Mortimer, 1983). Dementia is characterized by impairment in short-term and long-term memory, and at least one of the following: personality change or impaired judgment, abstract thinking, or higher cortical function such as aphasia, agnosia, or apraxia (Raskind & Peskind, 1992). Although there are exceptions, most dementias are insidious, progressive, and not reversible. The two most common types of organic dementias are Primary Degenerative Dementias of the Alzheimer's type (DAT) and Multi-Infarct Dementia. Distinguishing between normal aging and DAT, between depression and DAT, and between the subtypes of dementia have important treatment and prognostic implications (La Rue, Yang, & Osato, 1992).

The causes of Alzheimer's disease (AD) and subsequent dementia are receiving widespread attention. Among the multiple factors that might contribute to AD are genetic predisposition, abnormal protein synthesis, and environmental toxins (Raskind & Peskind, 1992). Multi-infarct dementias are thought to be related to repeated cerebral infarcts. Other frequent types are Parkinson disease dementia, affecting 10% of Parkinson's patients. Common to Alzheimer's disease and Parkinson's disease is depression, estimated to occur in 50% of patients with Parkinson's disease. AD's related dementias are progressive, although the course can be arrested with medication. Potentially reversible dementias include some metabolic dementias, such as those of hypothyroidism, repeated hypoglycemic episodes, or vitamin deficiencies, and some alcoholic dementias, most notably Wernicke's encephalopathy and Korsakoff's psychosis (McDougall, 1994; Raskind & Peskind, 1992).

Clearly, as the population ages, the number of individuals with dementias associated with aging will increase. If a quarter of older adults can expect to face dementia, health professionals must be prepared at the basic level to meet the demand these patients will make. In order to develop inpatient and outpatient systems to care for these patients, nursing education must incorporate knowledge and skills to support the acute- and long-term care of dementia patients.

The dementias and psychiatric disorders affect both cognitive and behavioral functioning. Among the areas for cognitive assessment are attention, concentration, intelligence, judgment, memory, orientation, perception, problem solving, psychomotor activity, reaction time, and social skills (McDougall, 1994). Activities of Daily Living (ADLs) such as dressing, grooming, toileting and bathing, and instrumental activities of daily living (IADLs), such as money management, taking medication, household maintenance, and communication (Fitzgerald, Smith, Martin, Freedman, & Wolinsky, 1993) also appear to be related to cognitive function. Functional ability has prognostic significance, serves as a gauge of both physical and emotional stability or decline, and is important to the caregivers since those with impairments can be encouraged to perform as fully as possible in all dimensions. Clearly, functional assessment of the older adult must be a part of any geriatric mental health educational program in nursing.

Delirium, in contrast, is a transient, usually reversible, acute confusional state that develops rapidly. These conditions of disrupted brain physiology, rather than the structural changes associated with dementias (Raskind & Peskind, 1992), are characterized by disturbances in consciousness. Episodes of delirium in the elderly are not uncommon and can be caused by infection, medication, metabolic changes, anesthesia, alcohol intoxication or withdrawal, or other physiologic, traumatic, and cardiovascular causes (Caine & Grossman, 1992). They are so prevalent that perhaps 50% of all elderly persons who are hospitalized experience these states. Early recognition by clinicians leads to prompt correction of the underlying disorder, underscoring the importance of the clinical competence in assessing these factors.

Treatment may include a range of therapies, including groups, remotivation, group and individual psychotherapy, life review, and memory training programs (McDougall, 1994). Older adults, once thought not to benefit from formal therapy, are responding well to therapeutic interventions. These interventions do not require all professional staff to have master's degrees, but basic preparation is essential for the therapists to be maximally effective.

Many elders with dementias are cared for at home by formal and informal, paid and unpaid caregivers. As Stommel, Collins, and Given (1994) note, the family costs of caring for patients with dementia are substantial. The incidence of depression and physical problems among caregivers is high (Drinka, Smith, & Drinka, 1987; Pagel, Becker, & Coppel, 1985), although adequate social support (Moritz, Kasl, & Berkman, 1989) and the use of faith or religion (Wykle & Segal, 1991) seem to be advantageous. In addition to treatment for patients, the caregivers require support. Groups such as the Alzheimer's disease support group require professional leadership. Therefore, a critical part of the geriatric mental health clinical student placement should include older adults in the community and their caregivers.

CLINICAL CONSIDERATIONS

The preconceptions and fears of students going into nursing homes about working with geropsychiatric patients is high. Such concerns should be dealt with early in the educational process, prior to clinical placement. Also, staff in facilities with mental health units tend to bias students in a negative manner toward older patients who may exhibit tenuous controls or unpredictable behavior. Sometimes mental health staff have difficulty accepting the chronic medical illnesses and functional disability that older adults may have. Students need to be prepared to handle these prejudices of peers as well. Prejudicial attitudes may be expressed as patronizing communications, less aggressive treatment approaches, and a tendency to stereotype the aged who have mental illness. Dealing with staff and student attitudes is essential. Most nursing homes are not expected to admit older adults with a mental illness unless they are able to adequately care for them. In a study of admissions to acute psychiatric units (Wykle, Segal, & Nagley, 1992) those depressed patients over age 70 had less aggressive care plans.

Although many older adults with mental illness are cared for in nursing homes, a substantial number of older adults with mental disorders, including cognitive impairments, receive short-term treatment in the general hospital setting (Kiesler & Sibulkin, 1987). The data of Keisler & Sibulkin indicate that approximately 30% of episodes of inpatient mental health care for elderly persons occur in general hospitals without psychiatric units, and that another 23% are treated in general hospitals with psychiatric units. Further, as many as 40%–50% of older adults hospitalized on medical-surgical units may have psychiatric disorders (Lipowski, 1983). Over the next decades, both nursing students and practicing nurses will encounter increasing numbers of older persons with geropsychiatric problems in all settings. A comprehensive geriatric mental health educational program is the cornerstone of providing progressive, holistic, and quality nursing care to older adults.

REFERENCES

Anthony, J., & Aboraya, A. (1992). The epidemiology of selected mental disorders in later life. In J. Birren, R. B. Sloane, & G. Cohen (Eds.), *Handbook of mental health and aging* (pp. 27–73). San Diego, CA: Academic Press.

Atkinson, R., Ganzini, L., & Bernstein, M. (1992). Alcohol and substance abuse disorders in the elderly. In J. Birren, R. B. Sloane, & G. Cohen (Eds.), *Handbook of mental health and aging* (pp. 515–555). San Diego, CA: Academic Press.

Berezin, M., Liptzin, B., & Salzman, C. (1988). The elderly person. In A. Nicholi (Ed.), *The new Harvard guide to psychiatry* (pp. 665–680). Cambridge, MA: The Belknap Press.

Blazer, D., Hughes, D., & George, L. (1987). The epidemiology of depression in an elderly community population. *The Gerontologist, 27*(3), 281–287.

Burns, B., & Taube, C. (1990). Mental health services in general medical care and in nursing homes. In B. Fogel, A. Furino, & G. Gottleib (Eds.), *Mental health policy for older Americans: Protecting minds at risk* (pp. 63–83). Washington, DC: American Psychiatric Press.

Caine, E., & Grossman, H. (1992). Neuropsychiatric assessment. In

J. Birren, R. B. Sloane, & G. Cohen (Eds.), *Handbook of mental health and aging* (pp. 603–641). San Diego, CA: Academic Press.

Drinka, T. J., Smith, J., & Drinka, P. (1987). Correlates of depression and burden for informal caregivers of patients in a geriatrics referral clinic. *Journal of the American Geriatrics Society, 35,* 90–117.

Erkinjuntii, T., Wikstrom, J., Palo, J., & Autio, L. (1986). Dementia among medical inpatients. *Archives of Internal Medicine, 146,* 1923–1926.

Evans, I., Funkenstien, H., Albert, M., Scherr, P., Cook, N., Chown, M., Hebert, L., Hennekens, C., & Taylor, J. (1989). Prevalence of Alzheimer's disease in a community population of older persons: Higher than previously reported. *Journal of the American Medical Association, 262,* 2552–2556.

Fitzgerald, J., Smith, D., Martin, D., Freedman, J., & Wolinsky, F. (1993). Replication of the multidimensionality of the activities of Daily Living Scale. *Journal of* Gerontology, *48*(1), S28–S31.

George, L., Blazer, L., Winfield-Laird, I., Leaf, P., & Fischbach, R. (1988). Psychiatric disorders and mental health service use in later life: Evidence from Epidemiologic Catchment Area program. In J. Brody & G. Maddox (Eds.), *Epidemiology and aging* (pp. 189–219). New York: Springer.

Gurian, B., & Goisman, R. (1993). Anxiety disorders in the elderly. In M. Smyer (Ed.), *Mental health and aging* (pp. 75–84). New York: Springer.

Haug, M., Belgrave, L., & Gratton, B. (1984). Mental health and the elderly: Factors in stability and change over time. *Journal of Health and Social Behavior, 25*(2), 100–115.

Jenike, M. A. (1989). *Geriatric psychiatry and psychopharmacology: A clinical approach.* Chicago: Year Book Medical Publishers.

Kiesler, C., & Sibulkin, A. (1987). *Medical hospitalization: Myths and facts about a national crisis.* Newbury Park, CA: Sage.

Koenig, H., & Blazer, D. (1992). Mood disorders and suicide. In J. Birren, R. B. Sloane, & G. Cohen (Eds.), *Handbook of mental health and aging* (pp. 379–407). San Diego, CA: Academic Press.

Krause, N. (1991). Stress and isolation from close ties in later life. *Journal of Gerontology, 46*(4), S183–S194.

La Rue, A., Yang, J., & Osato, S. (1992). Neouropsychological assessment. In J. Birren, R. B. Sloane, & G. Cohen (Eds.), *Handbook of mental health and aging* (pp. 643–663). San Diego, CA: Academic Press.

Lipowski, Z. J. (1983). The need to integrate liaison psychiatry and geropsychiatry. *American Journal of Psychiatry, 140*(8), 1003–1005.

McDougall, G. (1994). Mental health and cognition. In P. Ebersole & P. Hess (Eds.), *Toward healthy aging: Human needs and nursing response.* St. Louis, MO: Mosby-Year Book, Inc.

Moritz, D., Kasl, S., & Berkman, L. (1989). The health impact of living with a cognitively impaired elderly spouse: Depressive symptoms and social functioning. *Journal of Gerontology, 44* (1), S17–27.

Mortimer, J. (1983). Alzheimer's disease and senile dementia: Prevalence and incidence. In B. Reisberg (Ed.), *Alzheimer's disease: The standard reference.* New York: The Free Press.

Myers, J., Weissman, M., Tischler, G., Holzer, C., Leaf, P., Orvaschel, H., Anthony, J., Boyd, J., Burke, J., Kramer, M., & Stoltzman, R. (1984). Six-month prevalence of psychiatric disorders in three communities: 1980–1982. *Archives of General Psychiatry, 41,* 959–967.

National Institutes of Health Consensus Development Conference (Nov. 4–6, 1991). *Diagnosis and treatment of depression in late life.* Bethesda, MD.

Neugarten, B. (1969). Continuities and discontinuities of psychological issues into adult life. *Human Development, 12,* 121–130.

Pagel, M., Becker, J., & Coppel, D. (1985). Loss of control, self-blame, and depression: An investigation of spouse caregivers of Alzheimer's disease patients. *Journal of Abnormal Psychology, 94,* 169–182.

Rabins, P. (1992). Schizophrenia and other psychoses. In J. Birren, R. B. Sloane, & G. Cohen (Eds.), *Handbook of mental health and aging* (pp. 463–475). San Diego, CA: Academic Press.

Raskind, M., & Peskind, E. (1992). Alzheimer's disease and other dementing disorders. In J. Birren, R. B. Sloane, & G. Cohen (Eds.), *Handbook of mental health and aging* (pp. 478–503). San Diego, CA: Academic Press.

Regier, D., Boyd, J., Burke, J., Rae, D., Myers, J., Kramer, M., Robins, L., George, L., Karno, M., & Locke, B. (1984). One-month prevalence of mental disorders in the United States. *Archives of General Psychiatry, 45,* 977–986.

Sheikh, J. (1992). Anxiety and its disorders in old age. In J. Birren, R. B. Sloane, & G. Cohen (Eds.), *Handbook of mental health and aging* (pp. 409–429). San Diego, CA: Academic Press.

Stommel, M., Collins, C., & Given, B. (1994). The costs of family contributions to the care of persons with dementia. *The Gerontologist, 34* (2), 199–205.

Vogel-Sprott, M., & Barrett, P. (1984). Age, drink habits, and the effects of alcohol. *Journal of Studies on Alcohol, 45,* 517–521.

Wykle, M., & Musil, C. (1993). Mental health of older persons: Social and cultural factors. In M. Smyer (Ed.), *Mental health and aging* (pp. 3–18). New York: Springer.

Wykle, M., & Segal, M. (1991). A comparison of black and white family caregivers' experience with dementia. *Journal of the Black Nurses' Association, 5*(1), 29–41.

Wykle, M., Segal, M., & Nagley, S. (1992). Mental health and aging: Hospital care—a nursing perspective. In J. Birren, R. B. Sloane, & G. Cohen (Eds.), *Handbook of mental health and aging* (pp. 815–831). San Diego, CA: Academic Press.

Chapter 10

ELIMINATION AND SKIN PROBLEMS

Marie T. O'Toole

Incontinence, constipation, and skin problems are appropriate challenges to consider when planning educational programs for students of gerontologic nursing. The appropriateness of these topics, however, stems more from the need to correct misconceptions than a high priority need to consider these three problems as inextricably linked with the aging process. None of these problems represents the essence of gerontologic nursing and should not dominate the curriculum offerings related to the aging process. These topics can serve as a vehicle to illustrate a more accurate depiction of the needs of the older adult when woven throughout the curriculum. The focus of specific content on gerontologic nursing can then be a holistic presentation of the needs of the older adult and their family. Lack of time, competition with other specialities, and lack of interest are among the factors noted to be components that impede the inclusion of appropriate content in gerontology (Edel, 1986).

There are 31 million Americans over the age of 65 and individuals over the age of 85 are the fastest growing segment of the population (U.S. Department of Commerce, 1993), making it unimaginable not to educate students of nursing in components of vital aging. Moreover, our educational efforts should be directed toward achieve-

The author would like to acknowledge the insights and contributions of the nursing educators attending the session on elimination and skin problems and the group leader, Dr. Terry Fulmer.

ment of goals that are consistent with the contemporary nursing practice of health promotion and disease prevention. These goals should include avoiding problems with elimination and skin.

URINARY INCONTINENCE

Urinary incontinence is not a normal problem of aging. The causes of incontinence are complex, and can involve pathologic, anatomic, and physiologic factors that occur which are related to the urinary tract as well as factors outside it. Table 10.1 identifies some common causes of incontinence not directly related to the urinary system.

The normal physiologic change that occurs in the genitourinary tract as the individual ages can be divided into changes in the structure and function of the bladder, urethra, and in the male—the prostrate gland. The renal changes that can contribute to incontinence are most closely related to a decrease in the number of renal tubules that often results in an inability to concentrate urine. The end result of the loss of the ability to concentrate urine is a rate of urine production that does not vary over a 24-hour period and therefore contributes to urinary incontinence (Brundage, 1988). This type of information can be used in a nursing framework to develop a plan of care. It becomes a part of the analysis and should alert the student to the need to plan for toileting activities during the night. It is much more meaningful for a student to develop an understanding of a problem than to simply be presented with a solution.

The body of the bladder is lined with a smooth muscle called the detrusor. As individuals age this muscle can be replaced with fibrous connective tissue. Several problems may result: incomplete emptying of the bladder, decreased bladder capacity, and a decrease in the force of the urinary stream. Stress incontinence may occur when there is an increase in intrathoracic pressure such as that occurring when an individual coughs or sneezes. Urge incontinence is the involuntary loss of urine associated with an abrupt and strong urge to void. Urge incontinence is associated with involuntary detrusor muscle contraction, and is a common neurologic problem associated with a cerebrovascular accident (Urinary Incontinence Guideline Panel, 1992). Functional incontinence is caused by factors outside the urinary tract such as an inability to reach the toilet or commode due to a physical or cognitive impairment. With reminders of the physiologic base of some problems leading to incontinence the nurse should be encouraged to problem solve and use resources to assist the older individual to avoid incontinence.

It is important that students begin to develop an accurate expectation of the changes that can be anticipated with aging in introductory anatomy and physiology courses. A good understanding of the normal changes in the older client will allow the student to build a nursing assessment that is based on fact rather than myth. The proliferation of print and media advertisements for incontinence pads suggest that incontinence is both a universal and easily controllable problem associated with aging. Neither suggestion is correct. The percentage of individuals who are not hospitalized and are over the age of 60 who experience incontinence is 15%–30% (Merck, 1993).

The ability to control incontinence is based in large degree on the cause of incontinence. Overuse of urinary catheters is a contributing factor to the development of incontinence since this treatment exacerbates the loss of muscle tone. Clients who experience a loss of tone of the detrusor muscle are responding well to bladder retraining programs which usually incorporate the proper execution of Kegel exercises (Rose, Baigis-Smith, Smith, & Newman, 1990). Students should note that assessment of incontinence and a specific plan based on that assessment are necessary.

Educators should emphasize that these programs are often conducted by nurses. Students should be alerted to the role of the nurse with emphasis on the role of the gerontologic clinical nurse specialist in the care of older adults. The care of this individual is complex. This complexity will be best understood by the student when the nurse educator serves as a role model and frequently consults with colleagues possessing specialized expertise in problems affecting the older adult. The educator has the responsibility to familiarize the student with personnel and resource materials. An excellent resource for the assessment of individuals experiencing urinary incontinence is published by the Agency for Health Care Policy and Research and is entitled *Urinary Incontinence in Adults* (Urinary Incontinence

TABLE 10.1 Common Causes of Transient Urinary Incontinence

Potential causes	Comment
Delirium (confusional state)	In the delirious patient, incontinence is usually an associated symptom that will abate with proper diagnosis and treatment of the underlying cause of confusion.
Infection (symptomatic urinary tract infection)	Dysuria and urgency from symptomatic infection may defeat the older person's ability to reach the toilet in time. Asymptomatic infection, although more common than symptomatic infection, is rarely a cause of incontinence.
Atrophic urethritis or vaginitis	Atrophic urethritis or vaginitis may present as dysuria, dyspareunia, burning on urination, urgency, agitation (in demented patients), and occasionally as incontinence. Both disorders are readily treated by conjugated estrogen administered either orally (0.3–1.25 mg/d) or locally (2 g or fraction/d).
Pharmaceuticals	
Sedative hypnotics	Benzodiazepines, especially long-acting agents such as flurazepam and diazepam, may accumulate in elderly patients and cause confusion and secondary incontinence. Alcohol, frequently used as a sedative, can cloud the sensorium, impair mobility, and induce a diuresis, resulting in incontinence.
Diuretics	A brisk diuresis induced by loop diuretics can overwhelm bladder capacity and lead to polyuria, frequency, and urgency, thereby precipitating incontinence in a frail older person. The loop diuretics include furosemide, ethacrynic acid, and bumetanide.
Anticholinergic agents Antihistamines Antidepressants Antipsychotics Disopnamide Opiates Antispasmodics (dicyclomine and Donnatal) Anti-Parkinsonian agents (trihexyphenidyl and benztropine mesylate)	Nonprescription (over-the-counter) agents with anticholinergic properties are taken commonly by older patients for insomnia, coryza, pruritus, and vertigo, and many prescription medications also have anticholinergic properties. Anticholinergic side effects include urinary retention with associated urinary frequency and overflow incontinence. Besides anticholinergic actions, antipsychotics such as thioridazine and haloperidol may cause sedation, rigidity, and immobility.

TABLE 10.1 (*continued*)

Potential causes	Comment
Alpha-adrenergic agents Sympathomimetics (decongestants) Sympatholytics (e.g., prazosin, terazosin, and doxazosin)	Sphincter tone in the proximal urethra can be decreased by alpha antagonists and increased by alpha agonists. An older woman, whose urethra is shortened and weakened with age, may develop stress incontinence when taking an alpha antagonist for hypertension. An older man with prostate enlargement may develop acute urinary retention and overflow incontinence when taking multicomponent "cold" capsules that contain alpha agonists and anticholinergic agents, especially if a nasal decongestant and a nonprescription hypnotic antihistamine are added.
Calcium channel blockers	Calcium channel blockers can reduce smooth muscle contractility in the bladder and occasionally can cause urinary retention and overflow incontinence.
Psychological factors	Severe depression may occasionally be associated with incontinence but is probably less frequently a cause in older patients.
Excessive urine production	Excess intake, endocrine conditions that cloud the sensorium and induce a diuresis (e.g., hypercalcemia, hyperglycemia, and diabetes insipidus), and expanded volume states such as congestive heart failure, lower extremity venous insufficiency, drug-induced ankle edema (e.g., nifedipine, indomethacin) and low albumin states cause polyuria and can lead to incontinence.
Restricted mobility	Limited mobility is an aggravating or precipitating cause of incontinence that can frequently be corrected or improved by treating the underlying condition (e.g., arthritis, poor eyesight, Parkinson's disease, or orthostatic hypotension). A urinal or bedside commode and scheduled toileting often help resolve the incontinence that results from hospitalization and its environmental barriers (e.g., bed rails, restraints, and poor lighting).
Stool impaction	Patients with stool impaction present with either urge or overflow incontinence and may have fecal incontinence as well. Disimpaction restores continence.

Note: From Urinary Incontinence Guideline Panel. *Urinary incontinence in adults: Clinical practice guideline.* AHCPR Pub. No. 92–0038. Rockville, MD: Agency for Health Care Policy and Research, Public Health Service, U.S. Department of Health and Human Services, © March, 1992.

Guideline Panel, 1992). This resource includes sections that identify the use of the nursing interventions such as planning a time
voiding schedule, fluid intake control and biofeedback as well as
detailed models for the assessment of the client.

Aspects of this document are components of the evaluation and
management or urinary incontinence. Figure 10.1 demonstrates the
management model from this document. The message in class offerings regarding incontinence should be that it is always an abnormal finding and the cause of the incontinence should be fully assessed. Enlargement of the prostate in the form of benign prostatic
hypertrophy can cause an outlet obstruction and is a common cause
of urinary problems in older men. An enlarged prostate can cause a
dribbling of urine after urination, and frequency, nocturia and urgency
that can lead to episodes of incontinence. This specific problem is
important to introduce to students since it is estimated that as many
as 80% of men over 60 years of age experience this problem (Brundage, 1988). This particular problem helps to highlight the importance
of a thorough assessment. Other nonurinary causes of incontinence
include, but are not limited to, neurologic problems, malignancies,
and medications.

The social consequences of incontinence must be addressed and
its meaning for the older adult fully explored. Incontinence can serve
as a prototype for other preventable problems of aging that interfere with the quality of life for the older adult.

SKIN PROBLEMS

Skin problems in the elderly are caused by a variety of factors that
result in some obvious changes in the appearance of the older adult
There is a thinning of the epidermis along with collagen changes in
the dermal layer of the skin. These changes are responsible for the
loss of elasticity and the translucent appearance of the skin of most
elderly individuals. A loss of sebaceous gland activity results in dryness of the skin of individuals over the age of 70 (Matteson, 1988).
Vascularity of the skin is also reduced. A discussion of skin care of
the older adult presents the nurse educator with an opportunity to

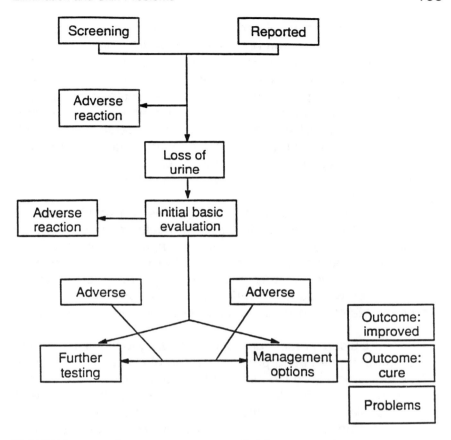

FIGURE 10.1 A management model for urinary incontinence in adults.

Note. From Urinary Incontinence Guideline Panel. *Urinary incontinence in adults: Clinical practice guideline.* AHCPR Pub. No. 92–0038. Rockville, MD: Agency for Health Care Policy and Research, Public Health Service, U.S. Department of Health and Human Services, © March, 1992.

encourage students to look beyond the obvious and explore the meaning of changes for the older adult. It is unlikely that the students will not recognize the importance of addressing changes in body image if given the opportunity to fully discuss the changes in the integument that inevitably accompany the aging process.

The student should also be encouraged to note the preventable nature of many problems related to the aging process. For example, when the effects of the sun on the integumentary system are presented it is important to emphasize that the pathologies associated with aging skin can often be eliminated by preventative care at earlier stages in life. Exposure to the sun, for example, is associated with a high incidence of skin cancers. The importance of health promotion throughout the lifespan can be strongly underscored by pointing out the links between behaviors and their sequelae in the later years. Special units to point out discrete pathologic problems are not needed to make the connection between health promotion and its beneficial effects.

An excellent example of integration of this content is illustrated by a discussion on burn injuries. As the faculty member presents material related to the prevention of burn injuries a reference can be made to the possibility of a severe sunburn resulting in a first- or second-degree burn, at any age. The long-term effects can be pointed out as well as the immediate danger burns present. Age-appropriate safety information can be interspersed throughout the discussion.

Pressure ulcers present another opportunity to highlight the role of the nurse in preventing problems in the older adult. Immobility, dietary deficiencies, and superficial trauma to the skin are all factors that play a role in the development of pressure ulcerations. These events, coupled with the changes in the skin described previously do place the older adult who is hospitalized at risk for pressure ulcers. When developing curricular materials, it would seem an ideal situation to encourage students to analyze the development of a pressure ulcer in an older adult. The analysis should lead to a recognition that immobility can be modified by the nurse through an individualized program of frequent range of motion, turning, and the provision of assistive and protective devices such as an overbed trapeze. Students should also be guided in the selection of appropriate assessment tools. For example, the Kenny Self-Care Scale is an excellent tool to use in a hospitalized older adult confined to bed. This scale incorporates bed activities such as independent turning, a definite advantage in both preventing pressure ulcers and encouraging behaviors that will encourage the client to be actively involved in care.

Nutritional deficiencies and superficial trauma also present opportunities to initiate nursing actions that clearly affect the development of pressure ulcers. The research literature is rich with examples that support the hypothesis that preventative nursing interventions affect outcomes related to skin integrity in the older adult. Requiring students to access this research base as they analyze skin care in the elderly also assists students to see issues related to the care of the older adult as integral to our nursing practice. It is strongly recommended that all nursing research courses incorporate reports addressing the nursing care of the older adult. Much in the same way that anatomy and physiology courses provide a foundation in the physiologic basis of changes associated with aging, research that addresses the nursing care of the older adult reinforces the nursing science foundation that is essential for quality care of the older adult, their family, and community.

Although it has been estimated that over 90% of older adults experience skin-related changes (Matteson, 1988), these changes need not be associated with pathology. Seborrheic keratoses, lentigos (liver spots), and xerosis (excessive dryness) are all very common disorders in the older adult. The student of nursing must learn to recognize these common problems and select nursing interventions that provide for both the comfort and safety of the older adult. Faculty in schools of nursing have a grave responsibility to select textbooks at all levels that adequately address the common changes that occur with the aging process. Most problems related to care of the skin in the elderly should be easily accessible to students in their fundamentals textbook. Additionally, the Agency for Health Care Policy and Research also provides an excellent resource entitled, *Clinical Practice Guidelines: Pressure Ulcers in Adults— Prediction and Prevention* (1992).

BOWEL ELIMINATION

Bowel elimination concerns are common in the older adult. Once again, the prevalence of the "problem" may overshadow the nature of concerns related to bowel elimination. As a consequence of re-

duced activity and changes in dietary patterns, most notably a reduction in the intake of fluid and fiber, there is often a reduction in
the number of bowel movements and a tendency of the stool to
become hard and dry. Constipation is a common, but not *expected*
finding associated with the aging process. Some medications that
are used frequently in an older population may also interfere with
normal gastrointestinal function. Once again, it is logical to point out
how well integrated content on issues that affect older adults can
become in the curriculum. Content on pharmacologic effects of the
gastrointestinal system can be easily incorporated into presentations
on classifications of drugs. Moreover, the focus should be broad—
the effect of all medications on the older adult should be noted—not
just the use or abuse of laxatives.

Students should be encouraged to assess the need for a bowel
program in any individual with a decrease in peristalsis or a neurologic problem that interferes with bowel function, not just the older
adult. A bowel program may or may not include a laxative. The design of a bowel program is highly individualized and must be reevalu-
ated on a continual basis (Association of Rehabilitation Nurses,
1994). The student should be reminded that drug interactions with
laxatives are not uncommon. Rehabilitation nurses can provide consultative services regarding the implementation of a bowel program.

The prevention of constipation will help to prevent the serious
problems associated with a fecal impaction. The student should be
aware of clients at highest risk for this problem (those on medications that result in diminished peristalsis, the immobile, unconscious
individuals, and individuals who have a past history of impaction).
The seriousness of a fecal impaction on the health of the older adult
can be incorporated into material that addresses critical care, a topi-
cal area that seems to quickly catch the attention and interest of
undergraduate students.

NEW THINKING ON ELIMINATION AND SKIN PROBLEMS

Consistently, throughout the discussion of the triad of problems that
are common in the elderly emerges the theme that students need

the background to distinguish between fact and myth in the older adult. A consensus has been reached that elimination and skin problems are not the most important issues in gerontologic nursing but rather represent barriers that often interfere with the education of students in vital aging.

In identifying content for nursing students in gerontologic nursing there needs to be a recognition that there are many essential guidelines that should be available to students as a resource. Concurrently, there should be an awareness that there is often a lack of knowledgeable faculty to assist the student in the interpretation of materials (Yurchuk & Brower, 1994), that text books often have little or no data on the aging process and focus on the consequences of problems rather than their prevention. This problem may grow in magnitude as the clinical nurse specialist is unavailable for consultation to both faculty and students. There is a concern that as hospital staffs are downsized, the absence of expertise and consultative services needed to adequately care for the older hospitalized adult will adversely affect outcomes of care. This reduction in nursing staff at an advanced level is a trend that should be carefully followed in the nursing research. There was a preexisting paucity of nurses prepared as experts in gerontology leading one to assume that the problem will be particularly acute.

The role of faculty who do possess expertise in gerontologic nursing is obvious; in addition to insuring that content is integrated throughout the curriculum the faculty must insure that gerontologic issues are highlighted. There should be a double-pronged approach that both develops a strong model of gerontologic nursing and also sensitizes colleagues to the need to address intergenerational issues at every opportunity. A colleague noted that the number of grandparents that are caring for young children has created the need to address learning styles of the older adult in content related to infants and newborns. There are numerous examples of active, noninstitutionalized older adults that can serve as excellent case studies in the curriculum. Yurchuck & Brower (1994) note that only 12% of undergraduate faculty in a regional survey had specific gerontologic preparation, but 94% of the faculty were interested in expanding personal knowledge of gerontologic nursing.

WAYS TO INFLUENCE POLICY

There is an old maxim in teaching that states, "You teach what you test." This can be expanded upon in this age when students are overwhelmed by the volume of material with which they are presented. They will study what is tested. The prevention of elimination and skin problems, as well as other problems in the older adult must be tested if they are to be mastered. Some test banks contain representative samples of issues that are related to the care of the older adult. Examples can be found in questions derived from Black and Martassarin-Jacob's Medical Surgical Nursing where a question on incontinence focuses on the psycho-social needs of the client (O'Toole & Bubb, 1993). Another important issue is to insure that questions from test banks, as well as questions authored by gerontologic faculty that address higher levels of cognition be included on the tests actually administered to the students. There are many helpful ways to track this information. One particularly helpful computer program called *Curriculum Manager* analyzes the questions entered into a computerized test bank in relation to curriculum objectives (Corbin, 1993). It not only provides an easy mechanism to create tests for students, but also gives faculty objective data as to how well (or if) they are measuring objectives with a pencil and paper examination. Essay questions also provide the opportunity for the student to interpret material.

The issue of testing usually raises the specter of the NCLEX-RN examination for the undergraduate student. It is reasonable to expect that the test pool includes a significant number of questions related to the care of the older adult. Faculty should nominate colleagues with expertise in gerontologic nursing to their State Boards of Nursing for item-writing activities. This single pro-active step signals a recognition that every nurse is called upon during their career to administer safe and effective care to the older adult. It is encouraging to note that the Board Review Book endorsed by the National Student Nurses Association, *NCLEX-RN Review* (Stein & Miller, 1994) includes a separate section entitled "Aging" that addresses care of the older adult, in addition to integration of material related to gerontologic nursing throughout other sections. This identification of a specific body of knowledge gives stature, similar to that which exists for pediatric or obstetrical nursing, to the essentials of safe care for the older adult.

Faculty should be mindful that curricula that contain organizing frameworks that move from birth to death and also incorporate a linear health–illness continuum can create the perception that aging= death and illness. Gerontologic nurse faculty must continue to contribute to the literature and identify journals whose readers would benefit from content related to care of the older adult. It is difficult to imagine an intensive care unit, a cardio-vascular unit, or rehabilitation unit that does not include older adults. Nurses working in these units should have access to information that enriches their knowledge of gerontologic nursing; they, in turn, serve as role models for the students during clinical rotations. The NICHE project (Nurses Improving Care to the Hospitalized Elderly) provides outlines for standards of care (Fulmer & Mezey, 1994), and is an excellent example of the information needed.

Ideally, every faculty will have an expert in gerontologic nursing among its members. In reality this is not the case at the present time and it is not likely to occur in the near future. This deficit can be addressed to some degree by continuing to utilize gerontologic textbooks and collaborating closely with clinicians involved in the care of older adults. It has also been suggested that transparency masters and other educational materials continue to be developed that address content in gerontologic nursing. There are outstanding educational videos that provide the nucleus for excellent class discussions of issues that nurses must address when caring for older adults. Conferences and references that identify essential content can also identify areas and strategies that insure adequate coverage of the content essential to the care of the older adult. *Teaching Gerontology: The Curriculum Imperative* (Waters, 1992) provides instructional strategies as well as excerpts from syllabi that are helpful. An important role we have as nurse educators is to inspire students to seek out roles where they can meet the needs of the older adult. When these students are ready for graduate study they will be more likely to seek specialization in gerontology.

The idea of "coverage" must not interfere with the current trend in nursing education of encouraging the development of critical thinking skills. Nosich (1994) notes that essential content is essential *for* something. Students need to be encouraged to master content on gerontologic nursing (including elimination and skin problems and their prevention) because they need to provide appropriate care to the older adult. Critical thinking helps students to reason through a problem in light of a clearly identified goal; the content provides a method for the student to achieve the goal. Caring for older Americans safely, with compassion and care, and addressing concepts of self-esteem and autonomy, are the overriding goals for nursing.

SUMMARY

Nursing educators face an important challenge as the number of older adults continues to grow. All students of nursing must have exposure to content addressing the needs of the older adult. Elimination and skin problems in the older adult can and should be fully explored, but they should serve as examples of preventable problems. The student nurse should be guided in the exploration of health promotion that builds on a solid scientific base. This is best accomplished by using a curriculum model that integrates themes that affect the older adult *and* by highlighting initiatives that promote healthy aging.

The absence of faculty with expertise in gerontologic nursing presents an obstacle in facing the challenge to incorporate gerontologic content in the curriculum but it is not an obstacle that is insurmountable. The availability of other nursing colleagues in the clinical setting as well as nurse educators who focus a portion of their practice on the care of the older adult provide resources on which to build. The development of educational resources, contributions to the nursing literature, and research in a wide variety of journals are expectations of faculty who are experts in gerontologic nursing.

There is content, and specific strategies to highlight content, identified within the body of this text. Nursing's goal and vision for the care of older Americans is what will guide our students. Our responsibility to help students keep that goal in mind should be the foundation of our curricular reforms.

REFERENCES

Association of Rehabilitation Nurses (1994). Core Curriculum in Rehabilitation Nursing. Skokie, IL. Author.

Brundage, D. J. (1988). Age related changes in the genitourinary system. In M. A. Matteson & E. S. McConnell (Eds.), *Gerontologic nursing* (pp. 280–289). Philadelphia: W. B. Saunders.

Corbin, S. (1993). *Curriculum manager-computer program.* Philadelphia: One on One HealthCare Productions.

Edel, M. K. (1986). Recognizing gerontologic content. *Journal of Gerontologic Nursing, 12*(10), 28–32.

Fulmer, T., & Mezey, M. (1994). NICHE Project. *Geriatric Nursing, 15*(3), 126.

Matteson, M. A. (1988). Age-related changes in the integument In M. A. Matteson & E. S. McConnell (Eds.), *Gerontologic nursing* (pp. 154–169). Philadelphia: W. B. Saunders.

Merck & Company (1993). *The healthy aging imperative.* West Point, PA: Author.

Nosich, G. (1994). Where to begin? How to design classes to teach for thinking. *Educational Vision, 2*(2), 20–22.

O'Toole, M. T., & Bubb, D. (1993). *Manual of test questions to accompany medical surgical nursing.* Philadelphia: W. B. Saunders.

Panel for the Prediction and Prevention of Pressure Ulcers in Adults. *Pressure Ulcers in Adults: Prediction and Prevention. Clinical Practice Guideline, Number 3.* AHCPR Publication No. 92-0047. Rockville, MD: Agency for Health Care Policy and Research, Public Health Service, U.S. Department of Health and Human Services. May 1992.

Rose, M. A., Baigis-Smith, J., Smith, D., & Newman, D. (1990). Behavioral management of urinary incontinence in homebound older adults. *Home Healthcare Nurse, 8*(5), 15–19.

Stein, A. M., & Miller, J. C. (1994). *NCLEX-RN review.* Albany, NY: Delmar Publishers.

Urinary Incontinence Guideline Panel. (1992). *Urinary incontinence in adults.* AHCPR Pub. No. 92-0038. Rockville, MD: Agency for Health Care Policy and Research, Public Health Service, U.S. Department of Health and Human Services.

U.S. Department of Commerce (1993). *Bureau of the Census, Current Population Reports, Special Studies, P23-178RV. Sixty-five Plus in America.* Washington, DC: U.S. Government Printing Office.

Waters, V. (1992). *Teaching gerontology: The curriculum imperative.* New York: National League for Nursing Press.

Yurchuck, E. R., & Brower, H. T. (1994). Faculty preparation for gerontologic nursing. *Journal of Gerontologic Nursing, 20*(1), 17–24.

Chapter 11

DRUGS AND THEIR SIDE EFFECTS

Barbara K. Haight and Karen Cassidy King

Nurses today enter a practice arena in which patients are older and taking multiple medications. In the adult population, 60 to 80 percent of clients across the continuum of care are over age 65, and increasingly over 85 years. Older persons over the age of 85 are the fastest growing segment of the older population (Waters, 1991). Currently, older people consume 25% to 30% of all prescription drugs (Sheahan, Hendricks, & Coons, 1989). Ray (1986) found that 61% of adults 65 to 84 living in the community (not in nursing homes or hospitals) received three or more different prescription drugs per year; 37% received five or more per year; and 19% received seven or more different prescription drugs per year. In nursing homes, the proportions were even higher. Thirty-four percent of 65- to 84-year-old residents received seven or more different prescription drugs (Ray, 1986). With the increasing aging population receiving multiple prescription and nonprescription medications, nurses need to have a broad knowledge base about aging, people, and medications.

Older people experience many physiologic changes where their first instinct is to reach for a pill. Many believe a doctor's visit is wasted if medication is not prescribed for a chief complaint. Over time, many older people accumulate a number of medications for a variety of reasons. Multiple chronic illnesses tend to encourage polypharmacy. Those with poor health status who have used large amounts of medications over time are most at risk for adverse drug reactions (ADRs).

In a survey of community-dwelling people age 65 and older, over 3000 people were asked to report ADRs. Ten percent of the sample reported one or more ADRs. For women, advanced age was associated with decreased risk, but a similar trend in men was not statistically significant. When the findings of this study were projected to the older community-dwelling population, ADRs accounted for 2.2 million annual physician visits, 1.1 million laboratory tests, and 146,000 hospitalizations (Chrischilles, Segar, & Wallace, 1992).

Noncompliance also contributes to ADRs in older people. Noncompliance is manifested in many ways and most acts are not deliberate behaviors to ignore the doctor's instructions. For example, noncompliance can result from thriftiness. Many older people cannot afford the prescribed medication and so attempt to stretch its use by taking it every other day instead of every day as ordered.

Noncompliance can also be a result of doctor shopping. Instead of returning to the family physician when a treatment is ineffective, the sick older person may seek out a second physician. They will then end up taking prescriptions from both doctors and potentially double dosing or having difficulties related to drug interactions.

Of course, there are many more common reasons for noncompliance. One major reason may be that the older person did not understand the directions for taking the medication in the first place and is too embarrassed to ask questions. They may not be able to read the written instructions or if it is time for hospital discharge, they may just be too overwhelmed by the many events surrounding discharge to be able to focus on instructions for taking medication.

Many researchers and educators have looked at ways to counteract nonadherence. Cargill (1992) examined the variables that influenced adherence and then used two levels of teaching interventions to influence medication compliance. She found that a follow-up telephone call caused a significant change in patient's risk-related behaviors. It was also very helpful to talk about the regimen and ascertain that there was congruence between the instructions and the taking of medications.

Another study distributed twice-daily medications to older outpatients in unit-dose packaging (Murray, Birt, Manatunga, & Darnell, 1993). To do this, the study group used geriatric outreach health centers in urban public housing units. Patients received one of three treatments: no change, conventional packaging, and/or a unit dose with all medications for a one-time dose contained in a 2-oz. plastic cup. Compliance was measured for 6 months using tablet counts. The group using unit-dose packaging were significantly more compliant than the other two groups. The authors concluded that elderly outpatients taking three or more medications will improve compliance if the medication is delivered in unit-dose packaging.

Older people do not really have a great deal of basic knowledge about medication. They trade information and may follow erroneous directions from friends who know only half of the story. O'Connell and Johnson (1992) conducted a study to evaluate medication knowledge in older patients. They asked people 60 or over taking more than one medication to recall their medications, tell what they knew about them, and report how compliant they thought they were. Thirty percent of the patients could name their medications and 27 percent always remembered to take their medications despite the fact that 86 percent of the sample said they never received oral or written instructions and only 27 percent were told of possible adverse reactions. So, the problem of noncompliance does not belong to the patient alone but also to those who prescribe and are responsible for patient education.

Inappropriate medication is a major cause of ADRs in older people. Lindley, Tully, Paramsothy, and Tallis (1992) examined 416 successive admissions to a teaching hospital. They found that interacting drug combinations and drugs with contraindications were commonly prescribed. Eleven percent of the admitted patients were taking drugs with contraindications, and immediately after admission, 175 drugs were discontinued because they were deemed not necessary. Of 151 ADRs, 75 were due to drugs that were unnecessary or absolutely contraindicated. The authors concluded that much of the drug morbidity in older people is due to inappropriate prescribing.

A similar study examined the potential for ADRs because of drug combinations. At least two-thirds of the respondents in this study reported drug/drug or drug/alcohol combinations that could be associated with ADRs when the medications are prescribed by the same physician (Pollow, Stoller, Forster, & Doniho, 1994). Of course, the physician has little control over the alcohol use of patients and alcohol/drug combinations can be as lethal as any drug contraindications. Most older people do not stop their medications when they drink, nor do they think of their alcohol intake as anything but social drinking.

Forster, Pollow, and Stoller (1993) looked at the frequency of alcohol consumption and concurrent use of medications in older community dwellers. They developed a profile of older drinkers and examined their clinical risk resulting from over-the-counter drugs, prescription drugs, and alcohol. Though 46 percent abstained from alcohol, those who did drink also took one or more drugs. The most common risk for drinkers was found in combining alcohol with over-the-counter pain killers.

One of the most significant treatable geriatric health problems is illness caused by medication. Aging people often experience drug induced depression (Ganzini, Walsh, & Millar, 1993). Drugs can also cause oral ADRs leading to taste changes, soft tissue reactions, and xerostomia (Lewis, Hanlon, Hobbins, & Beck, 1993). Poor sleep quality is related to drugs, particularly a history of the ingestion of sedative-hypnotic medications (Bliwise, 1992). Finally, neuropsychiatric reactions to drugs are also a problem for older people. The nonsteroidal antiinflammatory drugs cause neuropsychiatric reactions, particularly for females. They were, in fact, the third most common reported ADRs (Clark & Ghose, 1992).

BACKGROUND

What specific knowledge do nurses need in order to plan and provide quality nursing care to older adults? Nurses should be familiar with the pharmacokinetics, pharmacodynamics, and psychosocial factors associated with the use of medications in the elderly. It is imperative that nurses are taught to pay attention to dosage, monitoring, compliance, and drug interactions in the elderly population to prevent drug-induced illness and death.

Physical Considerations

Expected physical changes occur in the aging body that can influence the therapeutic effect of medications. The changes in physiology that affect medication use in older people are the result of either abnormal states that occur in older persons or normal age-related changes. The pharmacodynamics of drugs (the therapeutic effects of drugs at receptor sites) change because of the variation in individual aging and disease processes. Variation in pharmacodynamics occurs especially with diminished liver and kidney function, and results in unpredictable serum levels and half-lives of drugs (Beers, 1992).

The pharmacokinetic processes of absorption, distribution, metabolism, and elimination are altered by the physiologic changes of aging involving body composition and organ function. While the extent of drug absorption is not affected by age, few drugs have delayed rates of absorption after oral administration. Changes in body composition, protein binding, and blood flow do affect the concentrations of free unbound drug, the volume of distribution, and elimination half-life of a number of drugs. The primary goal of drug therapy in the elderly is to improve the quality of life. When medical therapy is required, the physician must be aware of the potential effect of age and disease on pharmacokinetics and pharmacodynamics and of the possible ramifications for ADRs or interactions. By increasing our knowledge of the action and effects of drugs in older people, and by enhancing communication and understanding between physician and patient, we can significantly improve the overall quality of care for the elderly patient (Williams & Lowenthal, 1992).

Absorption is the process by which drugs get from the external environment into the body, usually orally via the gastrointestinal tract. With aging however, gastric pH increases, absorptive surface decreases, splanchnic blood flow decreases, active transport decreases, and gastric acid secretion decreases (White, 1993). A decrease in absorption may occur in older people who have alterations in the gastrointestinal tract. However, this pharmacokinetic process is the least affected by aging. More important changes in absorption are caused by the simultaneous ingestion of several medications, which decreases the effectiveness of some and accelerates the effectiveness of others (Beers, 1992). Older people are more susceptible to the therapeutic and toxic effects of drugs.

Changes in body composition, plasma protein binding and blood flow alter the distribution of drugs; the process by which drugs move from the circulatory system to the tissues. Factors specific to the aging process that affect the distribution of drugs are decreased cardiac output, decreased total body water, decreased lean body mass and increased body fat (White, 1993). Elderly individuals with chronic liver failure, malnutrition, or renal failure can have severely decreased albumin concentrations.

Hepatic metabolism is the process by which a drug is converted chemically by enzymes in the liver. This enzyme action is responsible for biotransformation, or the conversion of drugs into metabolites enhancing drug metabolism (Oppeneer & Vervoren, 1983). Liver tests may be normal in the elderly even when all of the determinants of hepatic metabolism are significantly altered. Drugs that are eliminated primarily through liver metabolism have longer half-lives and reduced clearances. Age-related physiologic changes include decreased hepatic mass, decreased enzyme activity, and decreased hepatic blood flow. Liver disease, especially chronic liver failure, can lead to a decrease in clearance of some drugs metabolized by the liver (Wilkinson, 1986).

Drugs are typically excreted via the kidney into the urine or via the liver into the feces. The most predictable age-related pharmacokinetic change is the reduced rate of elimination of drugs by the kidneys (Knebl & Graitzer, 1994). Age-related changes include decreased renal blood flow, decreased glomerular filtration rate, and decreased tubular secretion. Normal renal function testing (BUN and creatine) does not reflect the actual renal function in older adults. Additionally, chronic diseases, such as hypertension, diabetic nephropathy, and congestive heart disease decrease renal excretion of medications (White, 1993).

Psychosocial Considerations

In addition to physical concerns, there are many psychosocial factors nurses need to consider with older people and medication management, including functional status, level of cognition, health beliefs, cultural influences, financial status, and education level. The overall functional status may affect the ability to read, to open medication bottles, to give injections if needed, or to adhere to a specific schedule. Level of cognition is equally important and can also affect the functional status. People with cognitive impairment tend to develop and rely on their social skills and are quite adept in hiding their deficiencies. They and their families may have little understanding of the inability of the cognitively impaired person to remember to take medications, or even to be able to sequence events in order to take them.

Health beliefs are another especially important influence and are different for all people. Building on the health belief model, the patient must believe the medication is going to help in order to be motivated to take it regularly. The nursing student needs to be able to assess and understand the patient's beliefs to help the patient comply. The medication must be important to the individual and the individual must want to take it. The nurse then must help the patient understand the importance of the medication.

Culture can also influence medication-taking and is closely related to health beliefs. For example, certain cultures believe in the hot/cold treatment of ills. A strep throat is hot. Followers of the hot/cold school would tend to treat the throat with crushed ice and throat spray. With this cultural belief system in place, it would be very hard to get the patient to take the necessary regimen of antibiotics. However, if the nurse understood the need of the patient to treat the strep throat in this way, the nurse could reinforce the hot/cold treatment while encouraging the patient to take antibiotics as well.

A social variable having a great impact on compliance is financial status. The earlier illustration of the person taking medicine every other day is a good indicator of the influence financial status has on a person's medication compliance. Conversely, some people who can afford the medication may think the price is outrageous and just not be willing to pay $1 a pill.

Educational level certainly can influence one's understanding of the medication regimen and the resulting compliance. Often the physician explains illness and treatment at a level above the average person's knowledge base. A poorly educated person, or one who cannot read, may have difficulty understanding complicated explanations.

NEW THINKING

Nurses need to engage in new ways of thinking to solve the problems of ADRs in older people. At a recent educational conference, a group of nurse educators brainstormed about teaching student nurses to handle some of these medication problems with older people. The group discussed necessary content, ways to present the content, and ways to influence policy in nursing education so that all nurse educators would appreciate the importance of the content in the curriculum. The group concurred that six major issues related to medication use needed to be included in the curriculum. Those six issues are listed in Table 11.1.

Psychosocial Issues

Psychosocial content should include family and caregiver issues. The student needs to understand the family as a system and recognize the issues created by the burden of caregiving in that system. Secondly, students must have an understanding of Alzheimer's disease and problems with cognition. They should be able to make an assessment of cognition and maintain an awareness of stages of cognition. People who are not cognitively intact are often incapable of

TABLE 11.1   Medication Content

1. Psychosocial Issues
2. Patient/Caregiver Education
3. Role of Nursing
4. Discharge Planning
5. Physiology
6. Drug Abuse and Misuse

being responsible for their own medication, though they nevertheless may be left with this responsibility.

Other psychosocial issues that students need to understand are the patient's belief and value systems and the impact of those systems on the patient's health. It is also necessary for students to know how much medicines cost and how much older people can afford to pay when they are receiving Medicare and buying medicine. Finally, students need to understand the patient's emotional makeup and coping ability. Each of these factors enters into a knowledge base necessary for the student to understand the older client's medication-taking practices.

Patient Caregiver Education

Patient caregiver education is another piece of information required by the student. The student needs to enhance the patient's understanding of the medication: how to take it, how to store it, how it works. The patient needs to be aware of the side effects and the possible interactions of their prescribed medication with other medications. The student should also be taught that the pharmacist is a ready and able consultant and available as a frequent resource. The student needs to explore how to educate using written or oral tools and how to recognize patient overload. The student also needs to know the difference between generic and brand name drugs, and relay all this information to the patient in a manner that will be understood.

Discharge Planning

Knowledge of discharge planning is imperative, especially knowing that it will begin on admission and that it is explicitly a nursing function. Discharge planning must be individualized and should use more than one route of delivering information. For example, some people learn best from oral input, others from written examples of information. It is therefore best for the nurse to explain medications and then to follow up with written directions for the patient to refer to at home. A chart that is color coded to color-coded medicine caps may also be helpful for the patient who cannot read well or who is illiterate.

Physiology

An understanding of physiological changes is essential to under-standing pharmacokinetics in older people. The nurse needs to understand age-related changes, the influence of nutrition and de-hydration, and disease interactions. Additionally, the nurse should be aware of changes in the drug transportation system, the drug's half-life, and the drug's action within the body. The nurse should also be familiar with vaccines and work to promote health and prevent disease.

DRUG MISUSE AND ABUSE

Drug misuse and abuse are important concerns. Medications have brand names and generic names that can cause the unintentional taking of duplicate medications. Multiple health care providers and the lack of coordinated care can cause unintended mediation duplication, while over-the-counter drugs can cause drug-drug interactions with other prescription drugs. A major contributor to the incidence of ADRs in the elderly is the inconsistent monitoring of drugs—prescription and over-the-counter—taken by older adults. The potential for drug inter-actions may increase as medications continue to be more readily approved for over-the-counter use. Approximately 30 percent of hos-pitalizations in the elderly are related to ADRs (Lamy, 1989).

Hoarding medications, drug sharing, and taking outdated medi-cations are behaviors that should be assessed. Education of the patient and caregiver are important nursing interventions to prevent drug mismanagement. Medication education should focus on proper drug storage, drug administration, drug actions, and possible adverse reactions with other drugs and with food.

Overutilization and underutilization of drugs is a problem in the elderly population. Polypharmacy places many older people at risk for developing ADRs. The more drugs an elderly person is taking, the less likely the individual is to take the drugs in the prescribed way. Many medications used for prevention and health promotion are underused. For instance, only 10 percent of older people have been vaccinated with the pneumococcal pneumonia vaccine and only 20 percent with the influenza vaccine (Williams, Hickson, & Kance, 1988).

Role of Nursing

Nurse educators must also plan the most efficient ways to teach this information to nursing students. Table 11.2 lists suggestions.

Teaching methods may be varied. Geriatric pharmacokinetics are the responsibility of the nurse and the pharmacist. An integrated module using both the expertise of the pharmacist and the nurse would add immensely to the student nurse's education. Such a module could be used in a basic educational program for nurses or in continuing education. A module designed for varied educational levels would make a strong inservice tool as well. Audiovisual aides have an added impact and should be incorporated into any educational plan because they have a strength that underlines the message. The future will also see growth in computer-assisted instruction, another aide for more intense education that should be freely used.

Finally testing, though threatening, is important. Many orientation programs require new employees to take a drug calculation test. This test should also contain information related to physiological changes associated with age to reinforce nurses' knowledge base and to help nurses realize what they need to know.

In addition to developing curricula that address medication issues among the elderly, nurses—especially nurse educators—

TABLE 11.2   Teaching Methods

1. Geriatric Pharmacy Module
2. Integrated Curriculum
3. Continuing Education
4. Inservice
5. Testing
6. Audiovisual Modules
7. Computer-Generated Instruction

must influence others to agree what should be done. One necessary step toward providing this knowledge base is to include content related to gerontology and pharmacology in nursing curricula. Content should include altered pharmacokinetics in the elderly, adverse effects of drugs in the elderly, nonprescription drug use, and polypharmacy. Content must be mandated by the National League for Nursing to be included in every accredited baccalaureate nursing program.

Finally, nursing educators must be advocates for the elderly. Nurses should support the policy that all clinical trials of drug metabolism, pharmacokinetics, and efficacy should include a reasonably sized sample of older subjects. Currently, the Federal Drug Administration does not require that the factor of age be considered when new drugs are tested. Recently, the pharmaceutical industry and the Federal Drug Administration have recognized the age bias in pharmaceutical research and now seek to include older people in clinical trials of drug efficacy and safety (Nightengale, 1991). An established standard should be set for drugs to be tested before they are put on the market.

Nursing has always been shaped by the population it serves. The knowledge and skills required for nursing practice have been determined by the clients under the care of nurses (Waters, 1991). Now is the time for nursing to realize that our aging clients have specific concerns with medications. Nursing curricula need to be reshaped to serve this growing population.

SUMMARY

Nurses must be knowledgeable about medications and the physiological and psychosocial changes of aging. They must also be mindful of the need to adjust doses for changes in pharmacokinetics and pharmacodynamics in the elderly. Drug-drug interactions should be noted, and medication histories taken frequently. Medication side effects should be considered with any change in function. Each of these important issues needs to be included in every nurse's basic education program.

REFERENCES

Beers, M. H. (1992). Medication use in the elderly. In E. Calkins, A. B. Ford, & P. R. Katz (Eds.), *Practice of geriatrics* (2nd ed., pp. 33–49). Philadelphia: W. B. Saunders.

Bliwise, N. G. (1992). Factors related to sleep quality in healthy elderly women. *Psychology & Aging, 7*(1), 83–88.

Cargill, J. M. (1992). Medication compliance in elderly people: Influencing variables and interventions. *Journal of Advanced Nursing, 17*(4), 422–426.

Chrischilles, E. A., Segar, E. T., & Wallace, R. B. (1992). Self-reported adverse drug reactions and related resource use. A study of community-dwelling persons 65 years of age and older. *Annals of Internal Medicine, 117*(8), 634–40.

Clark, D. W., & Ghose, K. (1992). Neuropsychiatric reactions to nonsteroidal anti-inflammatory drugs. *Drug Safety, 7*(6), 460–465.

Forster, L. E., Pollow, R., & Stoller, E. P. (1993). Alcohol use and potential risk for alcohol-related adverse drug reactions among community-based elderly. *Journal of Community Health, 18*(4), 225–239.

Ganzini, L., Walsh, J. R., & Millar, S. B. (1993). Drug-induced depression in the aged. What can be done? *Drugs Aging, 3*(2), 147–158.

Knebl, J., & Graitzer, H. (1994). Management of medications. In M. O. Hogstel (Ed.), *Nursing care of the older adult* (pp. 188–203). New York: Delmar.

Lamy, P. P. (1989). *Prescribing for the elderly*. Littleton, MA: PSG Publishing.

Lewis, I. K., Hanlon, J. T., Hobbins, M. J., & Beck, J. D. (1993). Use of medications with potential oral adverse drug reactions in community-dwelling elderly. *Special Care in Dentistry, 13*(4), 171–176.

Lindley, C. M., Tully, M. P., Paramsothy, V., & Tallis, R. C. (1992). Inappropriate medication is a major cause of adverse drug reactions in elderly patients. *Age and Ageing, 21*(4), 294–300.

Murray, M. D., Birt, J. A., Manatunga, A. K., & Darnell, J. C. (1993). Medication compliance in elderly outpatients using twice-daily dosing and unit-of-use packaging. *Annals of Pharmacotherapy, 27*(5), 616–621.

Nightengale, S. L. (1991). From the food and drug administration. *Journal of the American Medical Society, 265*, 182.

O'Connell, M. B., & Johnson, J. F. (1992). Evaluation of medication knowledge in elderly patients. *Annals of Pharmacotherapy, 26*(7–8), 919–921.

Oppeneer, J. E., & Vervoren, T. M. (1983). *Gerontology pharmacology.* St. Louis: Mosby.

Pollow, R. L., Stoller, E. P., Forster, L. E., & Duniho, T. S. (1994). Drug combinations and potential for risk of adverse drug reaction among community-dwelling elderly. *Nursing Research, 43*(1), 44–49.

Ray, W. A. (February 13, 1986). Prescribing patterns of drugs for the elderly. Conference Proceedings, *Pharmaceuticals for the elderly,* New research. Washington, DC: Pharmaceutical Manufacturers Association.

Sheahan, S. L., Hendricks, J., & Coons, S. J. (1989). Drug misuses among the elderly: A covert problem. *Health Values, 13*(3), 22–29.

Waters, V. (1991). *Teaching gerontology: The curriculum imperative* (Pub. No. 15–2411). New York: National League for Nursing Press.

White, C. P. (1993). Medications and the elderly. In D. L. Carnevali & M. Patrick (Eds.), *Nursing management for the elderly* (3rd ed., pp. 171–191). Philadelphia: Lippincott.

Wilkinson, G. R. (1986). Influence of hepatic disease on pharmacokinetics. In W. E. Evans, J. J. Schentag, & W. J. Jusco (Eds.), *Applied pharmacokinetics: Principles of therapeutic drug monitoring* (pp. 116–138). San Francisco: Applied Therapeutics.

Williams, L., & Lowenthal, D. T. (1992). Drug therapy in the elderly. *South Medical Journal, 85*(2), 127–131.

Williams, W. W., Hickson, M. A., & Kance, M. A. (1988). Immunization policies and vaccine coverage among adults: The risk for missed opportunities. *Annals of Internal Medicine, 108,* 616.

Chapter 12

Cancer and Pain Management for Elders: Recommendations for Nursing Curriculum

Suzanne K. Goetschius

ancer and pain management may seem like unlikely topics for a publication focusing on gerontological nursing education. Most nurse educators would recognize these topics as key content in their current curriculum. The question arises: Is there cancer and pain management content specific to the elderly that should be a part of a nursing curriculum? If so, why is it important? The prevalence of these two health problems among the elderly is significant. America is aging. As America ages, the resources necessary to deal effectively with cancer and pain management will be in demand. For a variety of reasons, the health care system is not adequately meeting the needs of these special groups of older adults. Nursing has the opportunity to respond to the challenges associated with the care and treatment of these two significant health problems. Some issues influencing the health care of elders with cancer and pain include the amount of inaccurate information considered true about aging and the older adult, the pervasive bias of ageism in both society and health care, the lack of an adequate theory base in these areas of gerontological nursing, and inadequate dissemination of the information that is available to assist nurses caring for older adults.

There exists a great deal of misinformation about aging and health in both the public and professional arenas. This leads to misconceptions and bias about health care and the older adult. The elderly are often the victims as well as the perpetuators of various myths of aging. An elder may believe that people are *supposed* to have pain as they age and not seek treatment for conditions such as arthritis. Perhaps even worse, a health care provider may respond to an elder's complaints with, "What do you expect at your age?" This may lead to a decrease in activity due to pain, perpetuating the stereotype of the older adult as disabled. It may lead to the delay in the treatment of a problem that will only be exacerbated by time. Elders may believe that a cancer diagnosis is equivalent to a death sentence and refuse to consider screening tests for cancer because they would "just rather not know."

Nurses can be prepared to intervene in cancer care and pain management to reduce disease and disability and increase the quality of life for elders. This can be accomplished through health education and health promotion activities. Nurses must also increase their understanding of and contribution to the specialized body of knowledge in gerontology in each of these areas to insure the competency and quality of the care they deliver. It is also important to examine the issue of ageism and begin to correct some of the inadequacies in the care of the older adult that exist as a direct result of the bias that exists against older patients. Nurse educators have the opportunity to introduce this information to nursing students. The National League for Nursing's (1993) vision for nursing education supports curriculum development in these areas.

BACKGROUND

Demographic data abound to illustrate the greying of America. The current predictions are that by the year 2030, 20% of the population will be over the age of 65 (AARP, 1993). This is a frightening statistic when it is correlated with the prevalence of cancer and pain in the older adult.

Age is the single leading risk factor for cancer. More than 50% of all cancers in the U.S. occur in persons over the age of 65. More than 60% of cancer deaths occur in the over-65 population (Kennedy, 1992). Commonly occurring cancers in the elderly currently include breast (female), lung, colorectal and prostate (Kennedy, 1992).

Many cancers are influenced by lifestyle factors such as diet, tobacco use, sun exposure or occupational exposure (Clark & McGee, 1992). Some cancers have an asymptomatic period during which currently available screening techniques can uncover the disease, allow for early treatment, and improve outcomes. Information about new treatment options reaches consumers through resources such as the media, support, and advocacy groups.

There has been a general decrease in the incidence of cancer among the population under the age of 55 (Erschler, 1992). Unfortunately for the population over the age of 55, the incidence of cancer continues to increase (Erschler, 1992). Despite the current available treatment options, prevention information, and screening techniques, older adults continue to experience significant disease and disability from cancer. Why does this occur and how can nursing improve this situation?

Older cancer patients often present with more advanced disease. This may be due to factors related to the older adult themselves, such as lack of information about their risk, lack of access to screening or avoidance, and delay in seeking treatment for health problems. Many elders have their own experiences with cancer or through a loved one; perhaps they witnessed great suffering and pain before death either because of treatment or the lack of it. Their fear of what they witnessed may prevent them from seeking treatment. Many women today fear mammography because of the stories they have heard about the test causing cancer or the pain caused by the breast compression needed to obtain an accurate examination (Clark & McGee, 1992). This may keep them from reminding their physician to schedule screening mammograms. Or, perhaps they are simply too embarrassed by the thought of having a rectal examination to bring up a new problem with constipation.

Health care providers may contribute to the prevalence of advanced cancer in the elderly. Paternalistic decisions to not "put the poor old dear through that uncomfortable exam" are made with good intentions but they rob the older adult of the opportunity to learn about the risks and benefits of the procedure and make an informed decision. Families may be involved in this as co-conspirators with the health care provider, protecting the older adult by not telling them about the recently discovered cancer. A variety of knowledge deficits exist between lay people, elders, and professionals that could be addressed through health education and health promotion activities by nurses with specialized knowledge about the myths and realities of aging and cancer.

Once a cancer is diagnosed, the elder will continue to face problems. Elders are at increased risk during the treatment phase for multiple reasons including their aging bodies, their diminished personal and financial resources, and ageism. The older adult is likely to have impaired bone marrow function and decreased renal function (Kennedy, 1992). These two age-related changes may predispose the elder to increased complications during chemotherapy. There are nursing interventions that can assist the elder at these times. The presence of comorbid illness and multiple medications may also cause problems during cancer treatment, but informed nursing assessment and critical thinking should help to reduce the incidence and severity of complications.

Ageism has had an impact on the research-based treatment of cancer. Many clinical trials which study antineoplastic therapy responses exclude the elderly from participation. Boyle (1994) states, "what has resulted is clinical decision making based on anecdotal and stereotypical information not necessarily formed in the patients' best interest" (p. 127). Nurses can begin to advocate for treatment based on sound research with elders if they are aware of these issues preventing the adequate treatment of older adults with cancer.

Elders also experience issues in cancer treatment related to psychosocial problems associated with aging. Limited financial resources are an issue for many older adults and may prevent the purchase of prescribed medication or food for adequate nutrition. Limited transportation may complicate follow-up treatment or a long radiation therapy course. An older adult may lack the emotional support of a spouse, family, or friends through loss, distance, or the multiple responsibilities of the caretaker today.

The nursing management of chronic and acute pain in the older adult is both a significant problem and a challenge. Elders are at increased risk for developing a chronic disease that leads to pain including arthritis, cancer, or diabetes. Elders may also experience acute pain superimposed on their chronic pain such as a hip fracture, postoperative pain, post herpetic neuralgia, or the pain of the progressing cancer. The incidence of multiple medication use, including over-the-counter drugs, in the older adult further complicates the management of pain in the elderly.

Ferrell, Ferrell and Osterweil (1990), found that the prevalence of pain in the nursing home resident is 70 percent. Crook, Rideout, and Browne (1984), learned that the prevalence of pain is two times greater in those over age 60 as compared to those under 60 in a survey of a general population. Although the knowledge is available to successfully manage up to 90 percent of pain, there is widespread undertreatment of pain by health care providers (Acute, 1992; Jacox et al., 1994). This undertreatment may affect the elderly even more because of the lack of knowledge that exists about pain management in the elderly, the lack of providers with specialized information about pain in the elderly, and the generalized ageism in health care.

There is little research available specifically related to pain in the elderly. Ferrell and Ferrell (1992), note that in over 5000 pages of gerontological nursing text, fewer than 18 pages addressed pain. These are the texts that are supposed to guide the care for the elderly? On the positive side, recently published guidelines for the management of acute postoperative pain and cancer pain each included sections related to the specific needs of the older adult (Acute, 1992; Jacox et al., 1994). The problems associated with nursing management of pain in the older adult can be attributed to ageism, myths and misconceptions, and inadequate knowledge of gerontological nursing.

As noted earlier, elders themselves may hold misconceptions about pain. They may view it as a normal part of aging. Untreated pain in the elderly may lead to decreasing activity levels, social isolation, or depression (Eland, 1988). Each of these problems may lead to further problems such as increased joint pain, loneliness, or loss of appetite.

Elders may hold misconceptions about the medications used to treat pain, particularly opioids. Like many people, they fear the possibility of addiction. Nurses are also prone to this fear that then leads to undermedication of patients in pain. Patients may fear that if they use opioids too soon during their disease, there will be nothing to relieve the pain at the end. Families may hold similar misconceptions. They may discourage the patient from taking pain medications to avoid addiction. They may be uncomfortable with the drowsiness that may accompany changes in medication.

Health care providers also have misconceptions about pain in the elderly. Many clinicians believe that pain thresholds increase with age although current data does not support this belief. Ferrell and Ferrell (1992) believe that this should not be a basis for treatment. Studies show that nurses believe elders cannot be treated safely with opioids because of the potential for respiratory depression (Brockopp, Warden, Colclough, & Brockopp, 1993; Ryan, Vorthems, & Ward, 1994). The incidence of respiratory depression in hospitalized adults receiving therapeutic doses of opioids is approximately 0.09 percent (Pasero & McCaffrey, 1994). Despite narrow therapeutic windows, many analgesic drugs can be used safely if the nurse is educated to assess the older adult accurately. It is key that nurses be able to use critical thinking skills in these situations to process and interpret the available information considering the multiple chronic health problems and medications that may characterize treatment of the older adult.

Accurate assessment of pain in the older adult can be difficult. This may be due to cognitive impairment or other health problems such as the pain itself, sensory impairments, or educational background, which may make it difficult to use some pain assessment tools. It may be necessary to do a mental status assessment before a pain assessment; if the elder is unable to participate in the assessment, the nurse must rely on other sources for assessment. For example, observation of the patient's behavior may reveal patterns that recur when the patient is in pain. Family members or significant others can contribute valuable information. There are many scales available to assess pain, and Herr and Mobily (1991) provide an excellent discussion of various pain tools.

Herr and Mobily (1991) identify factors that may impede the assessment of pain in the elderly. Beyond those reasons noted, the authors state that some patients may not report pain because of the fear of the consequences such as work-up of the complaint, loss of independence, or the expense. Not reporting pain may be a form of denial for some patients. Other patients use different terminology to describe their discomfort. Personal experience proved this fact one night while assessing a patient who was agitated, diaphoretic, and pale. When the patient was asked if he had chest pain he responded "no." A few minutes later the patient stated, "I'm not in any pain but I do feel like I have an elephant sitting on my chest."

Watt-Watson (1992) describes pain as a subjective experience determined by factors such as experiences with pain, the pain-producing situation, the anticipation of pain, the feelings of control, and cultural influences. Nurses often question the motives of people in pain, they may believe that the patient's complaints of pain may be an attention-getting mechanism. It is important for nurses to apply the old rule of thumb that all pain is real to the patient in pain. Emotional and psychological pain is just as real in the older adult as physical pain. Elders often suffer multiple losses including the loss of their support network. If the nurse believes the patient's complaints of pain are cries for attention, then the correct intervention may be to arrange for the patient to have this need met.

Current research shows that nurses consistently underrate their patient's pain or believe that patients overrate their pain (Camp, 1988; Rankin & Snider, 1984; Ryan, Vortherms, & Ward, 1994). Nurses may be undermedicating their older patients because of their fears about addiction or respiratory depression. Brockopp et al. (1993) note that knowledge deficits among nurses regarding pain are thought to result from inadequate education and lack of attention to this problem in practice settings.

NEW THINKING

In considering gerontology content for integration in a nursing curriculum it is important to consider both pain management and cancer content. Besides preparing students to better care for the needs of older adults, this content offers the opportunity to explore other issues in health care.

One example might be the impact of the media on the public's perception of health care issues. The death of comedian Gilda Radner focused much attention on the problem of ovarian cancer. Unfortunately, the public perception is that it is a disease of young women, when its peak incidence is in women age 55–59 (Clark & McGee, 1992). It is important for nurses to become involved in the education of the public through the media to assure the quality and appropriateness of the information delivered.

The focus of health education and health promotion of the elderly may have an impact on family and friends. If elders are caregivers for their children or grandchildren, it is important for them to have the appropriate information to pass along or to model. Elders may not derive much long-term benefit from the use of sunscreen today, but if they model this behavior and pass along the information, they may decrease the rate of skin cancer for future generations of elders.

Students must have a strong theory base if they are to develop critical thinking skills. This is especially true in gerontology where many problems are complicated by comorbid illness and poly-pharmacy. It is important for students to differentiate between normal aging and disease. For example, is constipation a part of normal aging or is it a warning sign of cancer? In the area of pain management, students must understand the changes in pharmacokinetics and pharmacodynamics that may impair the elder's ability to metabolize opioids. They must be able to assess mental status and the impact it may have on the assessment.

Ageism and the misconceptions that are part of both the health care delivery system and society should be examined and addressed. It is important for students to see elders outside of the institutional environment. Alternate sites that might provide appropriate learning opportunities include outpatient oncology or pain clinics, radiation oncology clinics, home health and hospice services, meal sites, senior centers, or social clubs. The student needs to demythologize their opinions about aging if they are to accurately assess and care for older adults.

It is also critical for students to be encouraged to include the older adult and their family in care planning. The elder is more likely to comply with the plan if they are involved in its conception. This simple act gives back to the elder a sense of control that can be particularly important to the patient with cancer.

It may also be important to the success of a plan to include the family. For example, a patient may begin a new medication regimen for pain that leaves them sleepy for the first few days. If family members are not included in this plan, they may see this as oversedation and try to scale back the medication, leaving the elder in pain.

Interdisciplinary approaches are important to the management of health problems in the older adult. Students should be encouraged to get involved in family team meetings, interdisciplinary rounds, and patient care conferences. An interdisciplinary team could also be useful in presenting the gerontology content to students. It might be possible to include students from other disciplines as well to reinforce the need to work collaboratively.

Students need to understand the variations in the nursing management of elderly patients undergoing chemotherapy, radiation, or surgery. The presence of cardiovascular disease, pulmonary disease, diabetes, or chronic renal failure may influence the elder's ability to tolerate treatment. Students should be tested on their ability to use critical thinking skills to evaluate the risks chemotherapy may hold for an older adult based on age-related changes in bone marrow function. Nurses must be aware of the alterations in pharmacokinetics and pharmacodynamics that accompany aging. Of particular concern is the incidence of drug-drug interactions related to changes in distribution. Changes in metabolism and excretion may affect dosages and the incidence of adverse drug reactions.

According to Boyle (1994), "The incidence and stages of cancer at diagnosis may be reduced if the elderly are targeted with intensive cancer screening and educational programs" (p. 132). Students may benefit by participating in cancer screenings and education programs. First, they should be exposed to the well elderly. Second, a screening may provide the opportunity to function as part of an interdisciplinary team. Third, depending on the type of activity, they should increase their knowledge of the assessment of older adults and cancer in the older adult. Fourth, they should learn about the process of providing health education to the older adult, and finally, educate the older adult about the role nurses can play in maintaining their health. It may also be beneficial to both staff and residents to have students involved in similar activities in long-term care facilities; such an experience will provide the student the opportunity to work with the frail elderly.

Students should be encouraged to explore service agencies and other care providers in their community to evaluate the accessibility, cost, and comprehensiveness of services available to older adults. For instance, what type of transportation service is available to elders who may need to attend radiation therapy five days per week for six weeks? Are services being duplicated? Does the pain management team make house calls? How does the home care agency handle the need to increase a patient's pain medication when the pharmacies are closed? This type of information could be shared with the class to increase the student's understanding of services and barriers to care for older adults.

Integrating content on cancer and pain management provides opportunities to examine issues common to nursing. The focus of caring versus curing is one that is central to the practice of gerontological nursing. The emphasis in gerontology is often on maximizing life and not postponing death. A clinical rotation for nursing students on an oncology unit provides the opportunity to discuss some issues nurses face when caring for patients who will die. One issue that often comes up is the impact of age on the nurse's sense of empathy for the patient. This serves as a starting point for discussions about topics such as treatment decisions based on age. For example, should an elder receive chemotherapy as a salvage or palliative procedure? What if the elder requests this type of treatment? Nurses often become involved in these types of ethical decision-making dilemmas. It may be beneficial to first explore these ethical dilemmas as a student.

Many ideas mentioned in this paper are examples of the curricular reforms called for by the National League for Nursing in *A Vision of Nursing Education* (1993). They recommend preparing nurses to function in a community-based health care system. Nurse educators are asked to assure that their graduates are competent in process skills such as critical thinking, collaboration, and analysis of health care systems. Curricular innovations include attention to the diversity of families and individual lifestyles and participative contact with consumers, especially those at risk. By integrating gerontology content as noted here, many of these reforms can begin to be addressed. More important, by preparing future generations of nurses to better meet the health care needs of the older adult, educators are serving the health care system. They are insuring quality care and preventing needless disability and suffering for older adults.

REFERENCES

Acute Pain Management Guideline Panel. (1992). *Acute pain management: Operative or medical procedures and trauma. Clinical practice guideline.* (AHCPR Pub. No. 92-0032). Rockville, MD: USDHHS, Public Health Service, Agency for Health Care Policy and Research.

American Association of Retired Persons. (1993). *A profile of older Americans: 1993* (AARP# D996). Washington, DC: AARP.

Boyle, D. M. (1994). Realities to guide novel and necessary nursing care in geriatric oncology. *Cancer Nursing, 17*(2), 125–136.

Brockopp, D. Y., Warden, S., Colclough, G., & Brockopp, G. W. (1993). Nursing knowledge: Acute postoperative pain management in the elderly. *Journal of Gerontological Nursing, 19*(1), 31–37.

Camp, L. D. (1988). A comparison of nurses' recorded assessments of pain with perceptions as described by cancer patients. *Cancer Nursing, 11,* 237–243.

Clark, J. C., & McGee, R. F. (Eds.). (1992). *Core curriculum for oncology nursing* (2nd ed.). Philadelphia: W. B. Saunders.

Crook, J., Rideout, E., & Browne, G. (1984). The prevalence of pain in a general population. *Pain, 2,* 49–53.

Eland, J. M. (1988). Pain management and comfort. *Journal of Gerontological Nursing, 14*(4), 10–15.

Erschler, W. B. (1992). Geriatric correlates of experimental tumor biology. *Oncology, 6,* 58–61.

Ferrell, B. A., Ferrell, B., & Osterweil, D. (1990). Pain in the nursing home. *Journal of the American Geriatric Society, 38*(4), 409–414.

Ferrell, B. R., & Ferrell, B. (1992). Pain in the elderly. In J. H. Watt-Watson

& M. I. Donovan (Eds.), *Pain management: Nursing perspectives* (pp. 349–371). St. Louis: Mosby-Yearbook.

Herr, K. A., & Mobily, P. R. (1991). Complexities of pain assessment in the elderly: Clinical considerations. *Journal of Gerontological Nursing, 17*(4), 12–18.

Jacox, A., Carr, D. B., Payne, R., Berde, C. B., Brietbart, W., & Cain, J. M. (1994). *Management of cancer pain. Clinical practice guideline No. 9.* (AHCPR Pub. No. 94-0592). Rockville, MD: USDHHS, Public Health Service, Agency for Health Care Policy and Research.

Kennedy, B J. (1992). Aging and cancer. In L. Balducci, G. Lyman, & W. B. Erschler (Eds.), *Geriatric oncology* (pp. 1–7). Philadelphia: J. B. Lippincott.

National League for Nursing. (1993). *A vision for nursing education.* New York: NLN.

Pasero, C. L., & McCaffery, M. (1994). Avoiding opioid-induced respiratory depression. *AJN,* April, 25–31.

Rankin, M., & Snider, B. (1984). Nurse's perception of cancer patient's pain. *Cancer Nursing, 7*(2), 149–155.

Ryan, P., Vortherms, R., & Ward, S. (1994). Cancer pain: Knowledge, attitudes of pharmacologic management. *Journal of Gerontological Nursing, 20*(1), 7–16.

Watt-Watson, J. H. (1992). Misbeliefs about pain. In J. H. Watt-Watson & M. I. Donovan (Eds.), *Pain management: Nursing perspectives* (pp. 36–58). St. Louis: Mosby-Yearbook.

Chapter 13

HIV AND OLDER ADULTS

Suzanne K. Goetschius

According to the World Health Organization (WHO) (1992), 30 to 40 million people worldwide will be infected with the human immunodeficiency virus (HIV) by the year 2000. This viral infection causes a general destruction of the immune system, leaving the infected person vulnerable to a multitude of opportunistic infections (OI) (El-Sadt et al., 1994b). The terminal manifestation of this infection is acquired immunodeficiency syndrome or AIDS. AIDS will be the third leading cause of death in the United States by the year 2000 (WHO, 1992).

Since the onset of the AIDS epidemic, there has been a stigma attached to being HIV positive, the societal tendency has been to point to a group of people and say this disease is their problem. Initially, AIDS was believed to be a disease of gay men and Haitians, later intravenous drug users were added to the list. Today it is recognized that HIV can infect persons of any sex, race, ethnic background, sexual orientation, or age. The mode of transmission of HIV is changing from predominantly homosexual contact to heterosexual contact. Women are now the fastest growing group of persons with AIDS in the United States (CDC, 1992), which will also affect the number of children infected and impacted by HIV. HIV will touch many families in every walk of life including the families of older adults.

The elderly as a population at risk for HIV infection has been ignored by the health care system. As a group, elders have not been the targets of educational programs, are unaware of their risk factors for transmission of the virus, are excluded from clinical trials for antiviral medications, and are rarely referred for HIV testing. Elders are not routinely talked about in nursing textbooks on HIV and yet nurses are frequently involved in the care of persons with HIV.

Nurses are the primary caretakers of older adults. Nurses have the opportunity to set the standard for the care of the older adult with HIV. Missing in nursing curricula is the distribution of information available about HIV and the older adult to student nurses. This chapter will help nursing faculty in the preparation of nurses skilled in the care of the elder with HIV. Compassionate caregivers are an important component of the management of challenging patients with difficult problems.

BACKGROUND

The older adult has been identified as comprising approximately 10 percent of all cases of AIDS (CDC, 1989). According to the CDC, there were 16,608 cases of AIDS in January 1991 in people over the age of 50. As of September 1993, there were now more than 34,000 persons with AIDS (PWAs) over the age of 50 (Geriatric Nursing, 1994). These statistics do not begin to address the numbers of elders who may have been infected and died before being tested or developing AIDS, the elders who died of AIDS but were never diagnosed, or those who are alive and unaware of their seropositive status. There are currently no seroprevalence studies among the elderly (Catania, Turner, Kegeles, Stall, Pollack & Coates, 1989).

Prevention of transmission is the most important means of controlling HIV in any age population until a cure or vaccine is discovered (Catania et al., 1989). Catania and colleagues note that development of an effective intervention to change behavior and prevent the transmission of HIV in a given population, there must first be a clear understanding of the pattern of transmission and the factors that influence that pattern.

The major mode of transmission of HIV in the older adult has been homosexual/bisexual contact (Ferro & Salit, 1992). Transfusion has been the second most common mode of transmission for elders, it is more common to the over-50 population who is more likely to have undergone transfusion in the period between 1978 and April 1985 when the blood supply was considered contaminated (Catania et al., 1989). Transfusion is an efficient mode of transmission but it may be limited to geographic areas where there are many possible HIV positive donors. Catania and colleagues noted that older individuals infected via transfusion may then infect others via sexual contact. They may not be aware that they received a transfusion, that they are seropositive, or that they can transmit the virus. Intravenous drug use (IVDU) was the third most common mode of transmission for the older adult followed by heterosexual transmission.

Catania and colleagues predict that the older adult may experience a significant but limited increase in HIV over the next five to ten years. This limited increase was based on the assumption that sexually active elders were in long-term monogamous relationships. The authors concluded, however, that the limits of HIV transmission in elders could not be defined because so little was known about the sexual activity of older adults. A study by Catania and Stall (1994) revealed that most of the new cases of HIV in older adults are a result of heterosexual transmission. The percentage of new AIDS cases attributable to heterosexual contact is greater among older Americans than any other age group. It is important for nurses to consider why elder transmission rates are increasing and what factors influence this increase.

One critical factor is that elders do not consider themselves at risk for HIV. Catania and Stall (1994) reported that 10 percent of older adults had at least one risk factor for HIV (number of sex partners, IVDU, hemophilia), but less than 7 percent had been tested for HIV and 85 percent never used condoms. These percentages were less than those of younger people with the same risk factors. A survey by Dawson (1988) noted that 84 percent of persons over age 50 believe they have no chance to get HIV; clearly a knowledge deficit exists.

The issue of sexuality in the older adult has significant bearing on the transmission of HIV in the older adult. The current cohort of elders was raised in an era when discussion of sex was a societal taboo. Elders may be unable to consider attending an educational program on HIV or asking questions of their health care provider. Nurses could have an effect in the development of materials to be used at home by elders. A survey by Gerbert and Maguire (1989) revealed that elders had read the Surgeon General's Report on HIV and AIDS, were glad that they had received it, and did not find it offensive.

Little data exists today to document the sexual practices of older adults. There is a persistent belief in society that elders are nonsexual and therefore, not at risk for HIV. The incidence of extramarital sex, sex with high risk partners such as prostitutes, the use of sexual aides and the sexual experiences of widowhood should be examined to help assess risk and guide educational programs (Catania et al., 1989).

Many stereotypes exist about sex and the older adult. The belief persists that elders are incapable of enjoying satisfying sexual relations because of physical deterioration, health problems, or lack of interest. The older adult may be sexually active throughout their seventies, eighties or nineties (Whipple & Scura, 1989). An elder who expresses interest in sex is often labeled a "dirty old man or woman." Elders may believe these myths, which can result in shame and guilt over their normal sexual desires. This shame and guilt may prevent them from admitting their sexual activity to health care providers. It may also prevent them from seeking information on sexual issues such as HIV or inhibit them from purchasing protective devices such as condoms.

Health care providers may also hold these ageist beliefs about sexuality and aging. They may not appreciate the risk of HIV transmission in older adults related to sexual practices or may be uncomfortable discussing sexual issues with the older adult. If they do not view the elder as having risk factors for HIV, they may not include them in health education planning.

They also may not encourage the testing of elders for HIV. The opportunity to begin early treatment of HIV and OIs may be missed if providers do not consider HIV as the potential differential diagnosis in older adults. Symptoms such as dementia, fatigue, lymphadenopathy, and atypical chest x-ray may suggest infection with HIV in the older adult. Nurses must also be aware of the risk of HIV infection in older adults as it relates to the practice of universal precautions. It would be hazardous to the health of a nurse if she/he assumed there was no need for universal precautions with older adults.

Social factors may lead to inadequate information or protection for sexually active elders. Elders living with their families may be embarrassed to express their sexual needs or lack the privacy necessary to meet those needs. Others may be without partners because of death or divorce and may be exploring options outside of a long-term relationship. Elders living in long-term care facilities may have their sexual activity restricted due to lack of privacy.

Nurses may be unprepared to facilitate the expression of sexuality among older adults (Quinn-Krach & Van Hoozer, 1988). The threat of HIV infection complicates the issue. There is a need to assure that safe sex occurs among elders and that elders have the information they need to protect themselves. If the nurse is responsible for insuring a patient's safety, then what role does the nurse have in preventing transmission of HIV among sexually active residents of long-term care facilities? Many issues are likely to be raised. For example, should condoms be offered? What about concerned families? Will the nurse feel comfortable teaching the elder to use condoms? What about elders with impaired dexterity for whom condom use may be difficult? Quinn-Krach and Van Hoozer (1988) recommend education to teach nurses to assess the sexual needs of older adults.

Testing for HIV in elders presents further issues for nurses. If elders do not believe themselves to be at risk for infection, they will not seek out testing. Many elders who have been tested did so because of transfusion notification programs (Catania et al., 1989). When testing does occur in elders, it is often at the request of a physician (Scura & Whipple, 1990). In one study, elders who were identified as having risk factors still refused testing despite their physician's request that they be tested (Catania, Stall, Coates, Pelham, & Sacks, 1989). Reasons that elders may not be tested include the stigma attached to the diagnosis of HIV and financial and access barriers that prevent testing. The poor rate of testing may contribute to the incidence of advanced disease at diagnosis among older adults (Ferro & Salit, 1992). El-Sadr et al. (1994b) report that, "early intervention and education often increase patient involvement in treatment, improve access to services, and slow the spread of disease" (p. 1). Without testing the older adult cannot benefit from early intervention and education.

The older adult may be at greater risk than young people for HIV due to changes in their anatomy and physiology. Studies show an increased rate of sexual transmission of infection with the increased age of the partner of the person with HIV (Catania et al., 1989). Changes in the vaginal mucosa related to decreased estrogen production is common in post-menopausal women. This may lead to breakdown of the vaginal wall and increase the opportunity for HIV transmission (Scura & Whipple, 1990). Changes in the immune system have been noted in the older adult (Catania et al., 1989; Ferro & Salit, 1992; Whipple & Scura, 1989) which may explain why elders have a shorter incubation time to AIDS.

Progression of HIV in older adults is different than in younger people. Data show that the time between transfusion with HIV infected blood to the diagnosis of AIDS is shorter in older adults than younger (Ferro & Salit, 1992); this holds true for other modes of transmission as well. Ferro and Salit noted the time from diagnosis to death was also shorter for older adults. Twelve percent of elders were likely to have an AIDS-defining disease at diagnosis as opposed to only 5% of those under age 40. The presence of comorbid illness such as chronic obstructive pulmonary disease, cardiovascular disease, cancer, or diabetes can decrease the elder's ability to endure opportunistic infections such as *pneumocystis carinii*.

The psychosocial trauma for the older adult with HIV may be more significant than for the younger adult. They will be the victims of bias against the old, and as they "live with the fear, pain and uncertainty of the disease, they also endure the prejudice, scorn and rejection by society" (El-Sadr et al., 1994b, p. viii). "Older adults with HIV may suffer more due to emotional isolation, absence of a support system and family tension. It can be a significant trauma for an older adult to reveal their HIV status to children or grandchildren" (AARP, 1988, p. 1).

HIV also affects elders as caregivers and as family members. "It has been estimated that about one-third of AIDS patients are dependent on an older parent for financial, physical and emotional support" (AARP, 1992, p. 1). This may be a heavy burden for some elders who may be receiving assistive services themselves or beginning their retirement. Even if the elder is not providing direct care to the PWA, they may be involved as caregivers for the children of PWAs. The care of a young child is a heavy burden compounded by the likelihood that the child may soon be orphaned or also be HIV positive.

Three related issues are important in assessing the caregiving burden. First, the elder must face the tragic realization that they will outlive their child or grandchildren. Besides the great emotional loss, the elder may have been counting on having the child or grandchildren to care for them as their health fails. Second, the elder may learn for the first time that their child is homosexual or has used intravenous drugs. This may lead to further isolation of the elder from their support network because of the stigma attached to these lifestyles by American society. Finally, the elder may need specialized information to teach their children or grandchildren to prevent further spread of the virus.

PWAs are living longer, requiring fewer hospitalizations, and are being managed on an outpatient basis as patients with a chronic disease (Hinkle, 1991). Financial concerns for families include the cost of health care, medications, and specialized treatments. Sometimes, the PWA may need specialized nursing care beyond the capabilities of the family to manage. Home care nurses are providing care to persons in the home with HIV and must be aware of the specialized needs of elders with HIV. Also, they may be providing services to the elder caregiver.

Linske, Cich, and Cianfrani (1993) note that between 10 and 25 percent of all cases of HIV may require long-term care services. There have been questions about the ability and willingness and the long-term care industry to meet this need. The authors found that some long-term care facilities were reluctant to consider HIV patients because of public relations issues, loss of private pay patients, reimbursement and the high cost of care for PWAS, fears and misconceptions of residents, families and staff, and the ability to protect the residents from infection. Facilities were more likely to consider an older adult with HIV or a resident who became HIV positive. They also noted that there was little request for long-term care beds for persons with HIV. Nurses in the long-term care field must begin to develop the expertise to care for the older adult with HIV.

NEW THINKING

Education of nurses to care for older adults with HIV must focus on the elder as patient and the elder as caregiver. It is important to begin with the stigma associated with HIV. HIV provokes a wide range of feelings in all people, including nurses. HIV curriculum is never simply an issue of testing, OIs, and medications. It often involves value judgments about alternate lifestyles, blaming the victim, fears of infection, and the futility of caring when death is inevitable. Nurse educators must be prepared to listen openly and nonjudgmentally to the concerns of students, especially the young, who may be examining these issues for the first time. Discussions of the bias that exists against persons with HIV and issues of ageism need to be addressed at the affective level (Eliason, 1993). The use of speakers, panels, and films including PWAs with follow-up small group discussion might ease this process (Eliason, 1993). In the clinical setting, a great deal of time must be allotted to processing feelings after clinical experiences involving PWAs.

It is important to begin with discussions about risk factors for transmission and the practice of universal precautions with all populations in all health care settings. Other critical content includes:

- the demographics of HIV in the older adult.
- physiologic characteristics of the older adult that may predispose them to infection.
- common myths and misconceptions about sexuality and aging.
- modes of transmission in the older adult.
- the dual stigma of ageism and AIDSism.

- presentation of HIV in the older adult (dementia, fatigue, adenopathy).
- lack of data on the safe use of antivirals in the older adult.
- incidence and prevalence of OIs and other manifestations in the older adult.
- impact on the older adult and their family.
- access issue, legal issues, financial issues and ethical issues in the treatment and care of older adults with HIV.

Some of the issues in the care of older adults with HIV are the lack of information the elders possess on HIV and the lack of data about the sexual activity of older adults. Many nurses have difficulty discussing sexuality with older adults. Students may benefit from examining some of these issues. For example, students can survey older adults about the risk for HIV among elders. The tool could be developed by the students to assess the issues relevant to their current focus such as prevention of transmission, elders beliefs about HIV, etc. The students should be given the opportunity to interview a well elder in a noninstitutional setting. This will serve to dispel the myth that all elders are frail and in hospital or long-term care settings. Students should be given content relevant to the discussion of sensitive topics with older adults such as sexuality in aging. Groups of elders could be reached at clinics, meal sites, senior centers, and various social groups. After the completion of the interviews, the data should be compiled and presented to the group for analysis. It would also be important to elicit the students' experiences in gathering the data; how they felt asking the questions, how did the elder respond, etc. The information presented earlier could be reinforced through roleplaying or review of individual situations.

Finally, after examining the data, the students should develop educational material to meet the assessed needs of the population they surveyed. Discussions about appropriate teaching methods with older adults would be important as would issues of cost, access and follow-up.

Another means for exploring the care of older adults with HIV would be to have students perform a community assessment of services. Service providers such as long-term care facilities, home-care agencies, and outpatient clinics could be assessed for access, educational background and experiences of staff, and issues they see in providing care to elders with HIV. Students could assess the amount of outreach to elders by resource and education groups, contact support groups to assess their experiences with elders as both patient and caregiver, and could explore access to the testing process for older adults. Discussions with local AIDS advocacy groups on legal and discrimination issues might be fruitful.

The delivery of comprehensive, compassionate care to persons with HIV requires a multidisciplinary approach (ANA, 1988). Nursing students should be exposed to this approach to assessment and care planning. Multidisciplinary teams of nurses, physicians, social workers, community educators, and others could present the necessary content and serve as a panel to discuss the issues relevant to care of the older adult. Students should be exposed to forums for collaborative care such as teaching rounds, team meetings, family meetings, and other multidisciplinary groups. The involvement of the patient and the caretaker in careplan development can not be over-emphasized. This is particularly important to the care of elders who may require the assistance of others, as may the PWA.

SUMMARY

Although homosexual/bisexual transmission still characterizes the majority of elders with HIV, the highest rate of increase of new HIV cases is among older heterosexuals. This may be due to sexual transmission by transfusees, lack of awareness among elders of their risk of sexual transmission), and the lack of effort toward educating a perceived "low-risk" group. The new awareness among providers that the elder is at risk for HIV infection may increase the rate of testing among this age group, resulting in the higher rate of newly reported cases. In addition, approximately 30 percent of PWAs may rely on their elder parents to provide physical care as their health declines.

Hinkle (1991) states that the implications for the nursing care of older adults with HIV include: "providing competent and compassionate care to clients with AIDS; developing a formal system of home-based health care tailored to the elderly AIDS patient; and educating colleagues and the general public to the facts of AIDS transmission and prevention" (p. 16). Nurses who are prepared to meet the needs of these challenging patients will be in demand since there is a lack of adequate treatment for HIV. Educators can assure a supply of nurses competently prepared to meet the needs of the elder with HIV by addressing the issues of ageism and AIDSism, exploring the current risk factors for HIV transmission in the elderly, discussing methods for teaching elders about HIV, and reviewing the anatomy and physiology of the older adult that predisposes them to problems with infection, treatment, and opportunistic infection. An added bonus would be the inclusion of research projects for students to examine the current state of elders' knowledge and the ability of the current health care system to meet the needs of the elder with HIV.

REFERENCES

Allers, C. T. (1990). AIDS and the older adult. *The Gerontologist, 30*(3), 405–407.

American Association of Retired Persons. (1988, June/July). Elderly and AIDS—Forgotten Patients? *Modern Maturity,* 17.

American Association of Retired Persons. (1992). AIDS: A multigenerational crisis (stock #D14942). Washington, DC: AARP/SOS.

American Nurses Association. (1988). *Nursing and the human immunio-deficiency virus: A guide for nursing's response to AIDS.* Kansas City, MO: ANA.

Catania, J. A., & Stall, R. (1994). AIDS risk behaviors among late middle-aged and elderly Americans. *Archives of Internal Medicine, 154,* 57–63.

Catania, J. A., Stall, R., Coates, T. J., Pelham, A., & Sacks, C. (1989). Issues in AIDS primary prevention for late middle-aged and elderly Americans. *Journal of the American Society on Aging, 13*(4), 50–54.

Catania, J. A., Turner, H., Kegeles, S. M., Stall, R., Pollack, L., & Coates, T. J. (1989). Older Americans and AIDS: Transmission risks and primary prevention research needs. *The Gerontologist, 29,* 373–381.

Centers for Disease Control. (1989, February 13). *AIDS weekly surveillance report.* MMWR. Atlanta, GA: CDC.

Center for Disease Control. (1992, July). *HIV/AIDS surveillance report.* Atlanta, GA: CDC. 3, 8.

Dawson, D. (1988). AIDS knowledge and attitudes for July, 1988, provisional data from the national health interview survey. *Advance Data from Vital and Health Statistics, 161,* 1–12.

Eliason, M. J. (1993). AIDS-related stigma and homophobia: Implications for nursing education. *Nurse Educator, 18*(6), 27–30.

El-Sadr, W., Oleske, J. M., & Agins, B. D., et al. (1994a). *Managing early HIV infection: Quick reference guide for clinicians.* (AHCPR Pub. No. 94-0573). Rockville, MD: USDHHS, Public Health Service, Agency for Health Care Policy and Research.

El-Sadr, W., Oleske, J. M., & Agins, B. D., et al. (1994b). *Evaluation and management of early HIV infections. Clinical practice guideline no. 7.* (AHCPR Pub. No. 94-0572). Rockville, MD: USDHHS, Public Health Service, Agency for Health Care Policy and Research.

Ferro, S., & Salit, I. E. (1992). HIV infection in patients over 55 years of age. *Journal of Acquired Immune Deficiency Syndromes, 5*(4), 348–353.

Gerbert, B., & Maguire, B. (1989). Public acceptance of the surgeon general's brochure on AIDS. *Public Health Report, 104,* 130–133.

Geriatric Nursing. (1994). AIDS affects older adults; guidelines released. *Geriatric Nursing, 15*(3), 121.

Hinkle, K. L. (1991). A literature review: HIV seropositivity in the elderly. *Journal of Gerontological Nursing, 17*(10), 12–17.

Linsk, N. L., Cich, P. J., & Cianfrani, L. (1993). The AIDS epidemic: Challenges for nursing homes. *Journal of Gerontological Nursing, 19*(1), 11–22.

Quinn-Krach, P., & Van Hoozer, H. (1988). Sexuality of the aged and the attitudes and knowledge of nursing students. *Journal of Nursing Education, 27,* 359–363.

Scura, K. W., & Whipple, B. (1990). Older adults as an HIV positive risk group. *Journal of Gerontological Nursing, 16*(2), 6–10.

Whipple, B., & Scura, K. W. (1989). HIV and the older adult: Taking the necessary precautions. *Journal of Gerontological Nursing, 15*(9), 15–19.

World Health Organization. (1992). *Global programme on AIDS: current and future dimensions of the HIV/AIDS pandemic.* Capsule Summary. Geneva, Switzerland: WHO.

Chapter 14

TEACHING ABOUT BIOETHICS AND THE ELDERLY

Mathy Mezey

In focusing on bioethical issues and the elderly, this chapter assumes that nursing students will have had exposure to basic content on bioethics. The recommendations in this chapter, therefore, are predicated on students being familiar with the fundamentals of bioethics, basic ethical theory, bioethical principles and methods, and on their having a working knowledge as to the relationship between bioethical and legal issues.

Nurse experts attending the conference, "Caring for Older Americans: The Critical Role of Nursing Education" spent several hours discussing bioethics and the elderly. There was consensus that all nursing students should have a working knowledge of bioethical dilemmas commonly encountered in geriatric practice. The following six points emerged from this discussion, coupled with a review of pertinent literature:

1. Students need opportunities to both identify and resolve bioethical dilemmas of actual older patients in the clinical setting. Teaching ethics in the classroom often leads to dissonance in the practice arena. Little learning will take place without providing students with opportunities to intervene in actual ethical dilemmas under the super-

vision of experienced faculty. Such experiences would strengthen students' skills in both advocacy and accountability.

2. Curricula should include content on both end-of-life decisions and the myriad of conflicts and ethical dilemmas that arise in providing daily nursing care to elderly patients. Examples of dilemmas include decisions about personal care such as feeding, management of disruptive behavior, and use of physical/chemical restraints.

3. While ethical dilemmas arise in the care of the "well" and younger elderly, the curriculum should reflect the most difficult dilemmas related to chronic illness, frailty, and the altered cognition seen with Alzheimer's disease, multi-infarct dementia, and strokes, especially among the very old.

4. Content should highlight assessment of decision-making capacity, including determination of decision-specific capacity.

5. Students need to gain an appreciation of the fact that often there are no easy solutions to bioethical dilemmas with the elderly, and that there is no "magic bullet" in resolving many dilemmas. Experiences should be structured to foster a degree of comfort with the ambiguity often involved in clinical decisions.

6. The values of patients, family members, and students/health-care providers, while always of importance in understanding decision-making, are of particular importance as they relate to geriatrics and long-term care. Emphasis should be placed on how the age, sex, ethnicity, race, class, and culture of students, health-care providers, the patient, and family members impact on bioethical decisionmaking.

PROTOTYPE CURRICULUM ON BIOETHICS
AS IT RELATES TO THE ELDERLY

In structuring the curriculum related to bioethics and the elderly, consideration should be given to the following components: (1) core didactic and clinical content on bioethics and the elderly that is required of all students; and (2) an elective course that offers students the opportunity to gain in-depth and individualized exposure, through both didactic content and a clinical practicum, to complex bioethical issues in care of the elderly. A third component of a model curriculum might also include an annual conference on bioethics and the elderly open to nursing students and other health-care professionals, and possibly offered for continuing education credits.

Required (Core) Content on Bioethics and the Elderly

There was agreement among the nursing experts as to the core geriatric content on bioethics and the elderly that should be compulsory for all undergraduate nursing students. The core includes both didactic content and clinical application. Topic areas to be included in such a core, as identified by nurse experts and the literature, include:

A. Determining decision-specific capacity in relation to informed consent and completion of advance directives. Decisions to agree or to forgo life-sustaining treatment for patients with and without advance directives; decisionmaking related to patients who lack decisionmaking capacity and have no written directives.

B. Ethical issues in the care of the elderly pertaining to the use of life-sustaining treatment.

C. Ethical issues in the care of the elderly pertaining to day-to-day care, including decisions related to feeding, toileting, bathing, decisions to hospitalize, use of physical and chemical restraints, decisions as to home and institutional care, and management of treatable conditions in patients with dementia.

D. Ethical issues related to enrolling cognitively intact, impaired, multicultural elderly in research studies.

E. Ethical issues related to resource allocation, including use of specialty units and costly treatments (dialysis, liver transplants, admission to coronary care units) in elderly patients.

For it to be effective, core content must be taught not only in the classroom but also in clinical rotations. This requires that faculty incorporate content related to bioethics and the elderly in seminars, pre- and post-conferences, and clinical rounds.

Nurse experts attenting "Caring for Older Americans" also spent considerable time discussing preparation of nursing faculty to teach both bioethics and geriatric nursing. There was general agreement that nursing faculty devalue both bioethics and geriatrics, and that avoidance of this content may, in large part, stem from ignorance and fear. Nursing faculty are perceived by these experts as fearing (1) the language of bioethics; (2) that they are unfamiliar with the "right" and "wrong" answers to ethical decisions; and (3) that they are not equipped to lead discussions concerning bioethical dilemmas, especially in small groups and in the clinical area.

Nurse experts reported a variety of strategies for creating a more receptive climate toward content in geriatrics and bioethics in the undergraduate curriculum, including involving faculty in research projects, fostering informal discussion of ethical dilemmas identified in newspapers and movies, and exposing faculty to experts in both geriatrics and bioethics. Existing resources, such as the Geriatric Education Centers (GECs) were seen as an untapped resource to help educate nursing faculty in geriatrics and bioethics.

An Elective in Bioethics and the Elderly

A bioethics course specifically relating to the elderly, including both didactic content and a supervised clinical practicum, should be offered as an elective for students wishing a more in-depth experience in bioethics. Such a course should be open to students representing several health professions. In some institutions, content in bioethics and the elderly might be offered as a certificate, for example, a training program in bio-ethics and values, which has been specifically developed to enable nurses, physicians, social workers, attorneys, pastoral counselors, and other professionals and selected scholars to undertake formal training in bioethics.

The basic geriatric content for such a course should focus on in-depth exploration of complex bioethical issues specific to the care of the elderly. This course would be drawn from, but not limited to content related to in-depth exploration related to decisionmaking capacity and end-of-life decisions, role of family members in decision-making for the elderly, ethical issues in the care of the elderly other than the use of life-sustaining treatment, and conducting research with cognitively intact and impaired elderly.

Experts attending "Caring for Older Americans" emphasized the need to teach models for ethical decisionmaking (Murphy; see others in Amidori), especially in the undergraduate curriculum. In most current nursing programs, undergraduate nursing students are taught to recognize ethical issues, but lack content and experiences in resolving dilemmas. Thus, students graduate feeling that most dilemmas are outside their realm of expertise and fail to understand their role in intervening and resolving dilemmas. Helping students use a decisionmaking model was seen as one way of increasing students' ability to intervene. Models would help students appreciate the complexity of decisions, mitigating their tendency to frame dilemmas in terms of black or white, and would emphasize the interdisciplinary nature in resolving ethical dilemmas in geriatrics.

Supervised observation of real dilemmas involving bioethical issues with the elderly in actual clinical situations should be a required component of an elective course. Personal contact between faculty and linking persons within health-care institutions was identified as one way of assuring that the clinical experience is based in reality. Another suggestion was to require students to maintain a log indicating where they or another staff member actually identified and acted on an ethical dilemma. Discussion related to the clinical experience could then focus on analyzing the decisionmaking and not just the dilemma.

The clinical practicum should be individualized and, where possible, include both interdisciplinary and discipline-specific experiences. Practicum opportunities could be developed in the home as well as in ambulatory, in-patient (including emergency rooms), and long-term care settings with strengths in bioethics, and/or governmental or voluntary agencies that deal with bioethical decisions.

When possible, didactic content should be delivered in small seminars that include lectures, case presentations, and discussion and role playing. Clinical practicums should include observations of such activities as ethics committees and ethics rounds, observational activities with patient representatives and social workers related to informing patients about advance directives, participation in ongoing projects and research related to bioethics and the elderly, and observational experiences with staff in agencies dealing with bioethical issues, such as choice in dying.

Evaluation of students who complete content in bioethics and the elderly should include written papers, class presentations, and class participation. Program evaluation should include: (1) completion of written student evaluations for all courses in the program; (2) interviews with students completing the courses; (3) written evaluations by faculty related to the content, student participation, etc.; (4) written evaluations by staff in collaborating clinical and other agencies.

Annual Conference on Bioethics and the Elderly

An annual conference open to a broad spectrum of university staff and health-care professionals, possibly offered for continuing education credits, would help to broaden the university and health-care community's exposure to issues related to bioethics and the elderly. Such a conference could draw on faculty involved in bioethics and the elderly courses, and should address relevant and timely ethical issues related to care of the elderly.

REFERENCES

Dubler, N., & Nimmons, D. (1992). *Ethics on call.* New York: Harmony Books.

Kane, R. A., & Caplan, A. L. (Eds.). (1990). *Everyday ethics.* New York: Springer.

La Puma, J., & Schiedermayer, D. (1994). *Ethics consultation.* Boston: Jones & Bartlett Publishers.

Lynn, J. (1989). *By no extraordinary means: The choice to forgo life-sustaining food and water.* Bloomington, IL: Indiana University Press.

Moody, H. R. (1992). *Ethics in an aging society.* Baltimore, MD: Johns Hopkins University Press.

New York State Task Force on Life and the Law. (1994). *When death is sought: Assisted suicide and euthanasia in the medical context.* New York: New York State Task Force on Life and the Law.

Veatch, R. M. (1989). *Cross-cultural perspectives in medical ethics: Readings.* Boston: Jones & Bartlett Publishers.

CHAPTER 14 APPENDIX
RESOURCES IN BIOETHICS AND THE ELDERLY

Resources within Colleges and Universities:
Philosophy departments
Institutional Review Boards
Humanities departments
Ethics committees
Schools of social work and law

General Resources:
The Georgetown University Center on Bioethics
Ethics Program—Harvard University
American Nurses Association
American Association of Critical Care Nurses
Geriatric Education Centers
Association of Nurse Attorneys
American Bar Association
Cultural advocacy groups
Gay advocacy groups
Organ donation groups

Videos:
AARP movie on ethics committees
Code Gray
AJN Interactive video
No Place Like Home.

Chapter 15

ON VITAL AGING[1]

Betty Friedan

I learned a lot from nurses in the ten years that I spent research-
ing my book, *The Fountain of Age*, including some things that doctors did not seem to know. I would like to give you a sense of the
paradigm shift with respect to age that I think that we as a society
are about to make and which will have profound implications for your
profession in dealing with older people. I would like to share with you
the sense that there is a mystique of age that is as pernicious, if not
more pernicious, more widespread, and harder to break through than
the feminine mystique was in the years before our new awareness
of "feminism."

Thirty years ago I wrote *The Feminine Mystique*, the book that
broke through the image of woman that everyone had accepted as
both conventional and sophisticated truth at the time: woman defined only in relation to man, woman as wife, mother, sex object,
housewife, and never a person defining herself by her own actions
in society. The image was everywhere, not only in women's magazines and on television, but in textbooks on sociology, marriage and
family—probably the textbooks you studied.

When I was fired from a newspaper job for being pregnant, I was
already feeling guilty that I was working, even though married to an

---

[1]This chapter is from a speech given by Betty Friedan at the "Caring for Older Americans" Conference,
held at the Grand Hyatt Hotel, New York City, January 6-7, 1994.

ex-GI in the theater and needing my paycheck. In that era "career woman" became a dirty word. The Freudian view that feminists were neurotics suffering from penis envy had wiped out of national memory the 150 years of struggle for women's rights. So I became a suburban housewife, writing for women's magazines like secret duty in the morning. No other mommy in that suburb worked outside the home. I wrote within the confines of the feminine mystique.

From a questionnaire of my Smith College sisters fifteen years after graduation and interviews of other suburban mothers I got a sense of a problem that had no name. The problem of these women had nothing to do with keeping the kitchen cleaned, ironing the husband's shirt, the children's bed-wetting, husband's ulcers, or the lack of the orgasm which defined the "women problem" then. This problem had to do with her own identity. "I'm B.J.'s wife, Jimmy and Janey's mommy, maker of beds, putter on of diapers, chauffeur, but who *am* I?" There was no word for the problem. I analyzed how we got to this point and put a name to the problem which helped bring about the change that your own careers have manifested: the personhood of women, with equal opportunity and a whole movement thereof. It changed the way our daughters looked at themselves as women and our granddaughters take it for granted. There has been a paradigm shift in the way women are viewed, in the way women view themselves, and in the possibilities of women's lives—and this shift changed everybody's lives.

A few years ago, I noticed another discrepancy between what everybody thought was true and what I was observing. I stumbled on it by accident. It started when I first looked for women who had moved beyond the feminine mystique. I interviewed women who were combining marriage, motherhood, and some profession beyond the home. At the time, it was an either/or situation, marriage-or-career, for many years in the feminine mystique era.

The women I interviewed in this regard were older than I was because my generation was still home bringing up the baby boomers. I discovered something interesting in passing. When I asked about menopause, then an unspeakable subject at the end of one's life as a woman, the answer again and again was, "Oh, I didn't have the menopause." Was I finding biological freaks? As it turned out, these women *thought* they hadn't had menopause because it was no big deal. They didn't take to their beds with depression, they weren't hospitalized for involutional melancholia (as many women were), and it was not the end of their lives as women. When real experience does not fit the book, my inner Geiger counter clicks. I consulted some of the medical experts in ob/gyn who insisted that some of the menopause was traumatic and that it did in effect mark the end of one's life as a woman. But I put the issue on the back burner because at the time I got involved in helping to start the women's movement. And somewhere in those hectic years I didn't have the menopause myself.

Robert Butler, who was head of the National Institute on Aging at the time, stated that he wanted to get me interested in age because most of the research and policy development on aging had been done by men, yet most of the people who are aged are women. Now this interested me as a feminist, except that I wasn't interested in age. I remembered the women I had interviewed who didn't have the menopause. I asked him was it possible that the way you define yourself as a woman and a person could actually have an effect on the biological process of aging, as it seemed to have had with these women'? And if so, what about men? It began to worry me that men were dying so much younger than women. I never did see the women's movement as a war against men. Women now have a life expectancy of nearly 86 years but for men it's now 72, and the difference has increased over the last century.

I thought there was something odd about this. Butler said that gerontologists didn't really deal with questions like that or had not yet asked those questions. So my inner Geiger counter decided that I was going to work on age. It was the hardest thing to do because I kept insisting that I wasn't *interested* in age. I had to work against my own denial the first few years I was working on the book.

I went to Harvard on a research fellowship to study aging, but in that whole big university the only work on the subject was at the medical school on Alzheimer's disease, nursing homes, and the ethical issues of when to turn off the machines. As I listened to the young Turks in white coats say things like "Do we give ourselves an unnecessary burden and worry too much about giving them a voice as to when to turn off the machine," it reminded me of many years earlier when I went to conferences on "the woman problem." Male experts on women would talk about "them." What can we do to get "them" off our backs, these frustrated, neurotic, suburban housewives that won't be content with PTA? Let's give them a basement room in the home-ec building for a continuing education course.

I searched for older people, like those first women I had studied, who defied the image of age. I thought they would be very rare because I accepted conventional beliefs about aging, just as in the beginning I had accepted the feminine mystique. I asked social workers and others in the community if they knew of any rare older individuals who seemed to be very vital, who continued to grow and develop, even thought they might not be Grandma Moses or Picasso. It turned out that these "rare individuals" were everywhere, even though at the gerontology conferences it was standing-room-only in the grand ballroom for presentations on incontinence in nursing homes and way down in the basement a workshop on creativity in later years was hardly attended.

I began to realize that there was a mystique of aging that defined age only as a process of deterioration and as a problem for society, not as what it is: a period of human life, a new period of human life at that. The life expectancy for women went from 46 years at the turn of the century to 80 now. There is a third to a half of life to which women can now look forward to and to which men should be able to look forward to as well, that is beyond youth and beyond menopause.

I was amazed to discover that, given the image of age as debility, only 5 percent of the elderly have Alzheimer's or any other kind of senility. That less that 5 percent are in nursing homes at any given time, and that only 10 percent ever will be. In recent massive studies done of women and men aging in their own homes, significant decline does not appear for most until well into their 80s (and that figure goes up every year), or just before death. The individual differences do not seem to be programmed for in this period of life; quality of life depends on what you do or do not do, or what society lets you do.

As the next part of my research I studied the mass media. I looked in magazines for pictures or illustrations or advertisements depicting those sixty-five or older. I could not find any, so I relaxed my standards and looked for anyone over fifty. One advertisement that I remember showed a rich and powerful-looking man draping a sable coat over the nude shoulders of a twenty-year-old bimbo. As for women, they were being sold everything and anything to deny age. Even advertisements for anti-age creams with names like "Youth Dew" or "Forever Young" featured an eighteen-year-old model with one line on her face. That research was done five or six years ago, but it is no different today. More recently the "waif" models seemed to shrink in those baby doll slip dresses as real women in America in all of their diversity of beauty got older. In all those magazines there was absolutely no image that was not "young," doing anything that any American would conceivably want to do—loving or arguing, winning or deciding something, playing, having fun, or just hanging out.

Yet the newspapers and magazines were more and more full of dreary stories about the "problem of age": the growing millions of people who "refused to die," the "fastest growing group" in the whole population, what is society to "do about the burden" of these poor, sick, senile, and unproductive older people on the "backs of the young"? Nearing that age myself, I was in a state of denial, which was obviously better than acceptance of what could be a self-fulfilling prophecy of age and decline. But denial is not a healthy state in American society.

As I got further and further into my book and began to think about the policy of walling older people off in adult playpens. Even when for the wealthy, these age ghettos in the middle of the desert are kept out of sight so as not to remind the rest of us that we are getting older. The focus of the discussion of age was on bored, sick people, while 95 percent of older people were not that at all. I began to look into the question of health care and I realized that we have to get beyond the denial. If you are going to say that "young is all," or "I'm 72 chronologically, but inside I'm 17," or "I'm forever 39," you buy the youth obsession. After the fifth facelift you don't look younger, you look inhuman. A man can shed this wife of forty years for a younger version and start all over again with babies. Now one even hears about 59-year-old women who want to have babies. I think they should have every right to, except that it *is* sort of foolish. We are free to look at this uncharted territory, the new third of human life beyond fifty, on its own terms with a sense of new possibilities and choices and meaning—for the personhood of age.

The first thing one has to do to come to this paradigm shift in regard to aging is to stop seeing older people only as objects of care, or age itself as sickness. When a patient comes to a doctor with some legitimate concern and the doctor says, "Oh well, that's just age," and prescribes some pills, it can lead to a hospital admission for over-medication. On the other hand, if the doctor does not want to look at this as a new period of human life, and treats older people as if they were young, that's denying age, which is almost worse.

Both in terms of my own interviews and others' research, we are just beginning to look at what happens when growth and development continues in these years, development that can not be measured by the yardstick of youth. People become more and more true to themselves and are less deterred by what other people have to say—they become truth-tellers, they become more whole. They can even be liberated from some of the things that drove and conflicted them in their youth and middle years.

This change has implications for health care; even senility is misdiagnosed when there is underlying depression. The depression that many older people suffer is understandable when you realize the conditions that exist for them. Older people are forced out of jobs, not only at 65 (even though that is supposed to be illegal now), but in their fifties with the downsizing of companies. Older people are made invisible in the community. They are taken seriously only as long as they can pretend to be young; once they are actually seen as old they are forced out of the mainstream and not taken seriously. This creates anger and depression that is inexplicable.

The paradigm shift involved in considering the personhood of age also involves a paradigm shift in care. Much of the medical debate on aging has focused on how too much money and too many medical resources are being spent on older people. It is not true that older people are sicker than younger people, but excess resources are perhaps condensed in the last weeks of life when expensive high-tech care is used to give women and men extra days of intractable pain and vegetative life beyond their own choices. Should not the goal be, rather than to shift resources from the old to the young, to maximize human function? What about vital old age? If there are limited health dollars should they be spent when the possibility of improving human function is nil, whether it be on premature babies or the last days of life?

I looked at what the research showed on what makes for a vital old age. Except for a few obvious things like smoking, the two main factors were purposes and projects to structure one's days and bonds of intimacy. In both cases these require staying in control of one's own life, retaining autonomy, staying in the community, being open to change, and being a part of change. The bonds of intimacy that people need in the later years are not necessarily the same as the childhood nuclear family or even youthful sexuality (which for men, the Kinsey study shows, peaks at age 17). Yet, intimacy remains a vital part of life in the older years. Purposes and projects are another matter if people are forced out of the community or forced out of productive work.

As far as health care is concerned, often the parameter of maintaining good care for people in the later years is not necessarily diagnoses and cure. The esoteric machinery of modern medicine is less important in these years than simply maximizing human function. The goal should be to make it possible for women and men in the later years to stay in control of their own lives and function in the community so that they can continue to live with purposes and projects and bonds that tie them into society. I was outraged to find nursing homes in which older people were not even called by their names, where excessive use of restraints and tranquilizers was common. The whole focus of health care should *not* be on nursing homes, but on keeping people functioning in their own homes, or new kinds of housing in the community.

I thought, when looking for vital older men and women, that the fountain of age, while it wasn't the fountain of youth, required breaking beyond the bond of youth to live longer and healthier lives. I found people recovering from strokes, heart attacks, and severe arthritis, who were vital and spirited. I met a woman who was teaching French to the other people in her retirement community (while recovering from a stroke). I was introduced to a wonderful psychiatrist who continued practicing until the very end of his life, who monitored his Parkinson's disease and kept a journal as he approached death.

In the last part of my book I talk about the freedom that comes with age, the sense that age can be an adventure, with freedom to invent new ways of loving and living, to invent a new self-image. The values that emerge in age can be different. Erik Erikson said that generativity is the opposite of stagnation and despair. In the case of older people, one has the opportunity to grasp one's whole life; its mistakes, tragedies, errors, triumphs, and realize that all of it is you. One is free to experience age as an adventure—and I do not mean trekking in the Himalayas—as a period of tremendous generativity. That is why it is so important that we stay in the intergenerational community, that our lives should be part of the stream of life that lives on after us, not only through our children and grandchildren, but through what you do. I have been struck by the examples I have found, of older people empowering each other and of their sense of obligation to the community. I love it when people plant trees that will not blossom until after they themselves have died. This generativity seems to he important as we move toward the big revolution of the personhood of age.

I cite some research in my book of a study in a nursing home in which some residents watered their own plants and some did not. Within a month, the residents who watered their own plants showed significant improvement in many of the indices of mental and physical health. After five years the people who took care of their plants were alive, while many of the others were not. This study makes an essential statement: that we must exercise our personhood, our human function—love, work, and choice.

Nurses are in a great position to be a part of the aging revolution. More than any other health professional, nurses already deal with the personhood of older people and sense that some of the important aspects of aging are not in the lesson plans of gerontology. As you begin to be even more adventurous in your own care of older people, you will develop even better ways to maximize function, control, and autonomy. Nurses who respect the personhood of age make efforts to maximize it. In recognizing that this takes precedence over diagnosis and cure, nurses can lead the revolution.

Appendix

Caring for Older Americans: The Critical Role of Nursing Education Conference

CONFERENCE COORDINATORS

Terry T. Fulmer, RN, PhD, FAAN
Professor of Nursing New York
  University, and Director,
  Columbia University-New York
Geriatric Education Center
New York, NY 10012

Cheryl Vince-Whitman
Vice President and Director
Health & Human Development
  Programs
Education Development Center, Inc.
Newton, MA 02158

ADVISORY BOARD

Mark H. Beers, MD
Associate Editor
The Merck Manuals
Merck & Co., Inc.
West Point, PA 19486

John R. Jezierski, MSN, RN
Director, St. Elizabeth Hospital
  School of Nursing
Lafayette, IN 47904

Mathy Mezey, RN, EdD, FAAN
Independence Foundation Professor
  of Nursing Education
New York University Division of Nursing
New York, NY 10012

Susan E. Sherman, MA, RN
Professor and Head
Department of Nursing
Community College of Philadelphia
Philadelphia, PA 19120

169

May Wykle, PhD, RN, FAAN
Florence Cellar Chair, Professor
  of Gerontological Nursing
Associate Dean

Frances Payne Bolton School
  of Nursing
Case Western Reserve University
Cleveland, OH 44106

PARTICIPANT LIST

William Abrams, MD
Merck & Co., Inc
West Point, PA 19486

Elaine Amella, GNP
Associate Research Scientist
New York University,
  Division of Nursing
New York, NY 10012

Barbara K. Andersen, EdD, RN
Associate Professor
The University of Tennessee
  at Chattanooga
Chattanooga, TN 37403

Amy Anderson, EdD, RN
Chair, Division of Nursing
Regis College
Weston, MA 02193

Doris Ballard-Ferguson, PhD, RNC
Associate Professor
University of Arkansas
  for Medical Sciences
College of Nursing
Little Rock, AR 72205

Cornelia K. Beck, PhD, RN
Associate Dean for
  Research & Evaluation
University of Arkansas
  for Medical Sciences
Little Rock, AR 72205

Linda Burnes Bolton, DrPH, RN, FAAN
Director, Nursing Research
  and Development
President, National Black
  Nurses Association
Los Angeles, CA 90048

Barbara J. Box, EdD, RN
Director and Associate Professor
Missouri Southern State College
Department of Nursing
Joplin, MO 64801

Linda Bucher, DNSc
American Association
  of Critical Care Nurses
Aliso Viejo, CA 92656

Mary Burke, DNSc, RN, CANP
Assistant Professor
Georgetown University
School of Nursing
Washington, DC 20007

Dr. Roberta Burris
Assistant Professor
Division of Nursing
University of Texas at Tyler
Tyler, TX 75799

Frieda R. Butler, RN, PhD, FAAN
Commonwealth Professor
George Mason University
College of Nursing and Health Science
Fairfax, VA 22030

Barbara Cammuso
Assistant Professor
Fitchburg State College
Fitchburg, MA 01420

Ann Carignan, MSN, RNC
Professor of Nursing
Valencia Community College-
  HPS Department
Orlando, FL 32811

Roberta Cavendish, PhD, RN
Professor
Wagner College
Staten Island, NY 10301

Helene M. Clark, PhD, RNC
Assistant Professor
The Catholic School of Nursing
Washington, DC 20064

Barbara Hassinger Conforti,
  MSN, RNC, CRNP
Instructor, Gerontology
Lancaster General Hospital,
  School of Nursing
Lancaster, PA 17603

Mary E. Coppola
Assistant Professor
Salem State College
School of Nursing
Salem, MA 01970

Pat deBoom, RN, MSN
Instructor, School of Nursing
Aurora University
Aurora, IL 60506

Rita DiCola
Assistant Professor
Alverno College
Milwaukee, WI 53234

Sister Rosemary Donley,
  SC, RN, PhD, FAAN
Executive Vice President
The Catholic University of America
Washington, DC 20064

Geraldine A. Evans
Chancellor
Minnesota Community College System
St. Paul, MN 55101

Marquis Foreman, PhD
Assistant Professor
University of Illinois at Chicago
College of Nursing
Chicago, IL 60612

Carolyn D. Foster
Curriculum Coordinator
Presbyterian Hospital School of Nursing
Charlotte, NC 28223

Catherine Taylor Foster
Nursing Department Chairperson
Southeast Missouri State University
Cape Girardeau, MO 63701

Eileen K. Gardner, EdD, RN
Assistant Professor and Chairperson
Department of Nursing
Jersey City State College
Jersey City, NJ 07305

Carol Gilbert, RN, PhD
Professor
Fitchburg State College
Fitchburg, MA 01420

Dr. Shirley Girouard, PhD, RN, FAAN
Executive Director
American Nurses Association, Inc.
Washington, DC 20024

Mary Tod Gray
Assistant Professor
East Stroudsburg University
East Stroudsburg, PA 18301

Jo Anne Grunow, DNSc
Assistant Professor
West Virginia University,
   School of Nursing
Department of Health Promotion/
   Risk Reduction
Morgantown, WV 26506

Dr. Sarah Gueldner
Director, Center for Nursing Research
Medical University of South Carolina
College of Nursing
Charleston, SC 29425

Dr. Barbara K. Haight, PhD, RN
Professor
Medical University of South Carolina
College of Nursing
Charleston, SC 29425

Patty Hannon
Assistant Professor
East Stroudsburg University
East Stroudsburg, PA 18301

Patricia Ann Hanson
Associate Professor,
   Department of Nursing
Nazareth College of Rochester
Rochester, NY 74618

Alene Harrison, EdD, RN
Chairperson, Department of Nursing
Idaho State University
Pocatello, ID 83209

Carol Heinrich
Assistant Professor
East Stroudsburg University
East Stroudsburg, PA 18301

Joseph J. Hill
President
Ralston House
Philadelphia, PA 19104

Jan Holloway, MA, RNC
Associate Professor
Intercollegiate Center
   for Nursing Education
Spokane, WA 99204

Susan R. Jacob, PhD, RN
Assistant Professor
Loewenberg School of Nursing
Memphis, TN 38152

J. Russell Johnson
Program Officer
The Pew Charitable Trusts
Philadelphia, PA 19103

Linda Kaeser, RN, PhD, FAAN
Professor, Isla Carroll Turner Chair
   in Gerontological Nursing
Director, Center on Aging
University of Texas–Houston
Health Science Center
Houston, TX 77030

Rose T. Kearney, PhD, RN
Director, Department of Nursing
Project Director, M.S.
   in Gerontological Nursing
ANE Program Grant
Department of Nursing
SUNY–College at New Paltz
New Paltz, NY 12561

Karen Cassidy King, RN, MSN, ARNP
Assistant Professor
School of Nursing
University of Louisville
Louisville, KY 40292

Muriel F. Kneeshaw,
  EdD, GNP, ANP, RNC
Associate Professor
College of Mount Saint Vincent
Riverdale, NY 10471

Erna Leslie
Columbia University School of Nursing
New York, NY 10032

Marianne K. Lettus, EdD, RN
Associate Dean, Nursing Programs
Regents College
Albany, NY 12203

Lois Malasanos, PhD, RN
Dean and Professor,
  Health Science Center
University of Florida
Gainesville, FL 32610

Carla Mariano, RN, EdD
Director, Master's Degree Programs
New York University
Division of Nursing
New York, NY 10012

Millie Marion
Assistant Professor
Fitchburg State College
Fitchburg, MA 01420

Joan Marren, RN, MS
Vice President for Clinical Service
VNS Home Care
New York, NY 10021

Miriam Martin, PhD, RN
Director
Goshen College
Goshen, IN 46526

Mary Ann Matteson, PhD, RN
Associate Professor, School of Nursing
University of Texas
  Health Science Center
San Antonio, TX 78284

Cheryl P. McCahon, MSN
Associate Professor, Nursing
Cleveland State University
Cleveland, OH 44115

Eunice C. Messler
Director, Nursing Program
Westbrook College
Portland, ME 04103

Linda Moran
Director, School of Nursing
Geisinger Medical Center
Danville, PA 17822

Phyllis K. More, PhD, RNC
Professor
Bloomfield College
Bloomfield, NJ 07003

Dolores A. Nelson, PhD, RN, MSN
Program Director, Associate Professor
Gannon University
Erie, PA 16541

Mary O'Donnell, MSN
Assistant Professor of Nursing
Community Health
Felician College
Lodi, NJ 07644

Marie O'Toole
Assistant Professor
Teachers College, Columbia University
New York, NY 10027

Elizabeth A. Parato, PhD, RN
Director of BSN Completion
Associate Professor of Nursing
Missouri Baptist College
St. Louis, MO 63141

Kathleen A. Peterkin
Assistant Professor
Alverno College
Milwaukee, WI 53234

Charon A. Pierson, RN, MS, GNP
Instructor/Coordinator FNP Program
University of Hawaii, Manoa
School of Nursing
Honolulu, HI 96822

Eileen J. Porter, PhD, RN
Associate Professor and Chair
Professional Program in Nursing
University of Wisconsin–Green Bay
Green Bay, WI 54311

Suzanne Fischer Prestoy, PhD, RN
Clinical Assistant Professor
Thomas Jefferson University
Quakertown, PA 18951

Joyce Rasin, PhD, RN
Assistant Professor
University of Maryland
  School of Nursing
Baltimore, MD 21201

Alice Redland, RN, PhD
Associate Professor
University of Texas at Austin
  School of Nursing
Austin, TX 78701

Sue Reed
Instructor, Nursing Division
Holy Family College
Philadelphia, PA 19128

Donna Regenstreif, PhD
John A. Hartford Foundation
New York, NY 10022

Veronica F. Rempusheski, PhD, RN
Nursing Administration
Beth Israel Hospital
Boston, MA 02215

Laura Robbins
Program Officer
John A. Hartford Foundation
New York, NY 10022

Janet A. Rodgers, PhD, FAAN
Dean and Professor
Philip G. Hahn School of Nursing
University of San Diego
San Diego, CA 92110

Evelyn L. Romano, RN
Associate Chief, Nursing Service
Department of Veterans Affairs
  Medical Center
Washington, DC 20422

Rosalie Rothenberg
Acting Dean, College of Nursing
SUNY Health Science Center
  at Brooklyn
Brooklyn, NY 11203

Dr. Sheila A. Ryan, PhD, RN, FAAN
Dean, School of Nursing
Director, Medical Center Nursing
University of Rochester
Rochester, NY 14642

Dr. Linda F. Samson
Acting Dean, School
  of Health Sciences
Clayton State College
Morrow, GA 30260

Shirlee Stokes
Associate Dean
Pace University
Pleasantville, NY 10570

Kathryn W. Sullivan, PhD, RN, CNAA
Professor
Research College of Nursing
Kansas City, MO 64132

Edith B. Summerlin, RN, PhD
Assistant Professor
University of Texas at Arlington
School of Nursing
Arlington, TX 76019

Jean Symonds
Associate Professor of Nursing
University of Maine, School of Nursing
Orono, ME 04469

Patricia Tabloski
Assistant Professor
School of Nursing
University of Connecticut
Storrs, CT 06269

Elaine Tagliareni
Assistant Professor
Community College of Philadelphia
Philadelphia, PA 19067

Mary P. Tarbox
Professor and Chair,
  Department of Nursing
Mount Mercy College
Cedar Rapids, IA 52402

Juanita Tate, RN, PhD
Associate Professor
University of Colorado,
  School of Nursing
Denver, CO 80262

Mary Tellis-Nayak
Director, Long Term Care
Joint Commission
Oakbrook Terrace, IL 60181

Saundra L. Theis, RN, PhD
Assistant Professor
University of Illinois College
  of Nursing
Chicago, IL 60612

Mary Ann Thompson, RN, MSN
Assistant Professor of Nursing
Saint Joseph College
West Hartford, CT 06117

Dr. Eleanor A. Walker
Associate Professor
Bowie, MD 20720

Lillian M. Waring, EdD, RN
Director, Health Science Division
Midwestern State University
Wichita Falls, TX 76308

Thelma S. Wells, RN, PhD
Professor
University of Rochester
School of Nursing
Rochester, NY 14642

Eleanor Wertz, MSN, RNC
Associate Professor, Nursing Division
University of Mary
Bismarck, ND 58504

Joan Zieja
Instructor, Nursing Division
Holy Family College
Philadelphia, PA 19128

INDEX

Abuse, of medications, 124–126
Accreditation process, incorporating geriatrics into the, 29–35
Acute care, issues in, 42
Advisory board, for conference, 169–170
Ageism
  awareness of, 53–55
  overcoming, in geriatric nursing education, 49–62
  practice issues, 55–58
  psychological aspects, 50–53
Aging
  anxiety disorders, 89–90
  bioethics and, core curriculum content, 155–156
  biological theory, 79–82
  changes, normal, and chronic illness, differentiation between, 82–83
  cognitive disorders, 92–94
  depression, 87–88
  frailty and, 15
  heterogeneity of population, lack of, reflection in geriatric nursing, 13–14

paranoia, 90
physiological changes in, 77–83
psychiatric disorders, 86–91
schizophrenia, 90–91
substance abuse disorders, 91–92
vitality in, 161–168
Alpha-adrenergic agents, as cause of transient urinary incontinence, 103
Annual conference, on bioethics and elderly, 158
Anticholinergic agents, 102
Antidepressants, 102
Antihistamines, 102
Anti-Parkinsian agents, 102
Antipsychotics, 102
Antispasmodics, 102
Anxiety disorders, and aging, 89–90
Assessment, psychological change, 81–82
Atrophic urethritis, as cause of transient urinary incontinence, 102
Awareness, of ageism, 53–55

177

B

Barriers, in geriatric nursing
    education, 21–28
Benztropine mesylate, 102
Bioethics, and elderly
    annual conference on, 158
    core curriculum content,
        55–156
    elective in, 156–158
    geriatric nursing, 153–159
    prototype curriculum, 154–158
    resources in, 159
Biological theory, of aging, 79–82
Bodily elimination, 99–114. *See*
    Elimination
Bowel elimination, 107–108

C

Calcium channel blockers, as
    cause of transient urinary
    incontinence, 103
Cancer, in elderly, 129–140
Caregiver education, about
    medications, 123
Changes, in aging, normal, and
    chronic illness, differentiation
    between, 82–83
Channel blockers, calcium, as
    cause of transient urinary
    incontinence, 103
Chronic illness, and normal aging
    changes, differentiation
    between, 82–83
Clinical practice, in geriatric
    nursing, 37–47
    advanced, preparation for, 8–10
    beginning, preparation for, 4–8

Cognitive disorders, aging, 92–94
Community nursing, geriatric
    nursing education, 41–42
Conference, annual, on bioethics
    and elderly, 158
Conforti, Barbara Hassinger, 171
Confusional state, as cause of
    transient urinary
    incontinence, 102
Coordinators, of conference,
    169–170
Core curriculum content, bioethics
    and elderly, 155–156
Course-specific programs, *vs.*
    integrated, in geriatric
    nursing education, 63–66
Curriculum for geriatric nursing
    education, 3–19, 4–12, 16,
    37–47, 39–40
    accreditation process,
        incorporating geriatrics into
        the, 29–35
    acute care, 42
    ageism, overcoming, 49–62
    barriers in, 21–28
    bioethics, 153–159
        elective in, 156–158
        prototype curriculum,
            154–158
    bodily elimination, 99–114
    cancer, 129–140
    clinical practice, 37–47
        advanced, preparation for,
            8–10
        beginning, preparation for,
            4–8
    clinical sites, alterative, 40–43
    community nursing, 41–42
    course-specific programs, *vs.*
        integrated programs, 63–66

faculty, 39–40
  preparation of, 16
  requirements, 45–46
frail elderly, 15
gaps in knowledge, 10–11
graduate clinical training sites, 43
graduate students, 44
HIV, 141–152
home health care, 42
intergenerational issues, elderly
  elderly, failure to address, 14
Kellogg, W. K., Nursing Home
  Partnership Project, 70–73
licensure process, incorporating
  geriatrics into, 29–35
long-term care, 42
medications, side effects of, 115–128
mental health clinical
  experiences, 44–45
models, 67–74
  development, 12–13
  interdisciplinary education, 15
  medical, 58–60
pain management, 129–140
physiological changes, in aging, 77–83
prototype, bioethics and elderly, 154–158
psychiatric mental health
  content, 85–98
Robert Wood Johnson Teaching
  Nursing Home Project, 69–70
side effects of medications, 115–128
skin problems, 99–114

students, 38–39, 40–43
  undergraduate, 45
vitality, in aging, 161–168

D

Decongestants, as cause of
  transient urinary
  incontinence, 103
Depression, and aging, 87–88
Dicyclomine, as cause of
  transient urinary
  incontinence, 102
Discharge planning, medications, 123
Disopnamide, 102
Diuretics, 102
Donnatal, 102
Doxazosin, 103

E

Education, in geriatric nursing. *See
  also* Geriatric nursing
  education
  barriers in, overview, 21–28
  state of, overview, 3–19
Elderly. *See* Aging
Elective, in bioethics and elderly, 156–158
Elimination, 108–109
  geriatric nursing, 99–114
  urinary incontinence, 100–104
Emotive aspects, of ageism, 50–53
Excessive urine production, as
  cause of transient urinary
  incontinence, 103

F

Faculty
  and curriculum issues, 39–40
  curriculum issues, 39–40
  preparation of, 16
  requirements for, 45–46
Focus, gerontological nursing,
    5–6
Frail elderly, 15

G

Geriatric nursing
  focus, 5–6
  model, 12–13
  preparation, 5–6
  work overview, 5–6
Geriatric nursing education, 37–47
  accreditation process,
      incorporating geriatrics into
      the, 29–35
  acute care, 42
  ageism, overcoming, 49–62
  barriers in, 21–28
  bioethics, 153–159
    elective in, 156–158
    prototype curriculum, 154–158
  bodily elimination, 99–114
  cancer, 129–140
  clinical practice, 37–47
    advanced, preparation for,
        8–10
    beginning, preparation for,
        4–8
  clinical sites, alterative, 40–43
  community nursing, 41–42
  course-specific programs, *vs.*
      integrated programs, 63–66

curriculum, 39–40
  gaps in knowledge of, 10–11
  intergenerational issues,
    elderly, failure to address,
    14
  models, 67–74
faculty, 39–40
  preparation of, 16
  requirements, 45–46
frail elderly, 15
graduate clinical training sites,
    43
graduate students, 44
HIV, 141–152
home health care, 42
Kellogg, W. K., Nursing Home
    Partnership Project, 70–73
licensure process, incorporating
    geriatrics into, 29–35
long-term care, 42
medications, side effects of,
    115–128
mental health clinical
    experiences, 44–45
model
  for interdisciplinary education,
    15
  medical, 58–60
overview, 3–19, 4–12, 16
pain management, 129–140
physiological changes in aging,
    77–83
psychiatric mental health
    content, 85–98
Robert Wood Johnson
    Teaching Nursing Home
    Project, 69–70
side effects of medications,
    115–128
skin problems, 99–114

students, 38–39, 40–43
undergraduate students, 45
vitality, in aging, 161–168
Graduate clinical training sites,
  geriatric nursing education,
  43
Graduate students, geriatric
  nursing education, 44

H

Heterogeneity of elderly
  population, lack of reflection
  of, in geriatric nursing,
  13–14
Hill, Joseph J., 172
HIV, 141–152
Home health care, 42
Human immunodeficiency virus
  See HIV, 141–152
Hypnotics, sedative, as cause of
  transient urinary
  incontinence, 102

I

Illness, chronic, and normal aging
  changes, differentiation
  between, 82–83
Impaction, stool, as cause of
  transient urinary
  incontinence, 103
Incontinence, urinary, 100–104
  transient, causes of, 102–103
Infection, urinary tract,
  symptomatic, as cause of
  transient urinary
  incontinence, 102

Integrated programs, *vs.* course-
  specific programs, in
  geriatric nursing education,
  63–66
Interdisciplinary education, models
  for, 15
Intergenerational issues, elderly
  elderly, failure to address,
  14

L

Licensure process, incorporating
  geriatrics into, 29–35
Long-term care, 42

M

Medical model, geriatric, 58–60
Medications
  abuse of, 124–126
  discharge planning, 123
  patient caregiver education, 123
  physical considerations, 119–120
  physiology, 124
  psychosocial issues, 120–123
  side effects of, 115–128
Menopause, symptoms of,
    absence of, in vital aging
    women, 162–163
Mental health, 86
  geriatric nursing education,
    85–98
  clinical experiences, 44–45
Misuse, of medications, 124–126
Mobility, restricted, as cause of
  transient urinary
  incontinence, 103

Model
  curriculum, geriatric nursing
    education, 67–74
  for geriatric nursing, 12–13
  for interdisciplinary education,
    15
  Kellogg, W. K., Nursing Home
    Partnership Project,
    70–73
  medical, geriatric, 58–60
  Robert Wood Johnson Teaching
    Nursing Home Project,
    69–70

N

Nursing curriculum. *See also*
    Curriculum
  heterogeneity of elderly
    population, lack of reflection
    of, 13–14
Nursing programs, geriatric. *See*
    Geriatric nursing

O

Opiates, as cause of transient
    urinary incontinence, 102

P

Pain management, geriatric
    nursing education, 129–
    140
Paranoia, aging, 90
Participant list, for conference,
    170–175

Patient caregiver education,
    medications, 123
Pharmaceuticals, as cause of
    transient urinary
    incontinence, 102. *See also*
    Medications
Physical considerations,
    medications, 119–120
Physiological change, in aging,
    77–83
  normal, functional results of,
    80–81
Physiology, medications, 124
Policy, influencing, 110–112
Practice issues, in ageism, 55–58
Prazosin, as cause of transient
    urinary incontinence, 103
Preparation, gerontological
    nursing, 5–6
Prototype curriculum, on bioethics,
    and elderly, 154–158
Psychiatric disorders, and aging,
    86–91
Psychiatric mental health content,
    geriatric nursing education,
    85–98
Psychological change,
    assessment of, 81–82
Psychological factors
  of ageism, 50–53
  as cause of transient urinary
    incontinence, 103
Psychosocial issues, medications,
    120–122, 122–123

R

Resources, in bioethics and
    elderly, 159

Restricted mobility, as cause of transient urinary incontinence, 103
Robert Wood Johnson Teaching Nursing Home Project, 69–70

S

Schizophrenia, aging, 90–91
Sedative hypnotics, as cause of transient urinary incontinence, 102
Side-effects of medications, use in geriatric nursing, 115–128
Skin problems, 104–107, 108–109
Stool impaction, as cause of transient urinary incontinence, 103
Students, geriatric nursing education, 38–39, 40–43
Substance abuse disorders, and aging, 91–92
Sympatholytics, incontinence, 103
Sympathomimetics, incontinence, 103
Symptomatic urinary tract infection, incontinence, 102

T

Terazosin, as cause of transient urinary incontinence, 103
Transient urinary incontinence, causes of, 102–103

Trihexyphenidyl, and benztropine mesylate, as cause of transient urinary incontinence, 102

U

Undergraduate students, geriatric nursing education, 45
Urethritis, atrophic, as cause of transient urinary incontinence, 102
Urinary incontinence, 100–104
transient, causes of, 102–103
Urinary tract infection, symptomatic, as cause of transient urinary incontinence, 102
Urine production, excessive, as cause of transient urinary incontinence, 103

V

Vaginitis, as cause of transient urinary incontinence, 102
Vitality, in aging, 161–168

W

W. K. Kellogg, Nursing Home Partnership Project, 70–73
Women, and menopause, absence of symptoms, 162–163
Work overview, gerontological nursing, 5–6